A Life
of
Caring

16 NEWFOUNDLAND
NURSES TELL THEIR STORIES

Marilyn Marsh ❧ Jeanette Walsh ❧ Marilyn Beaton

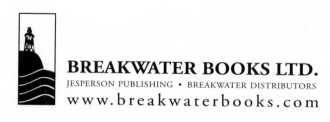

BREAKWATER BOOKS LTD.
JESPERSON PUBLISHING • BREAKWATER DISTRIBUTORS
www.breakwaterbooks.com

Library and Archives Canada Cataloguing in Publication

Marsh, Marilyn, 1932-
    A life of caring : sixteen Newfoundland nurses tell their stories
    Marilyn Marsh, Jeanette Walsh & Marilyn Beaton.

ISBN 978-1-55081-251-0

1. Nursing--Newfoundland and Labrador--History. 2. Nurses--
Newfoundland and Labrador--Biography. I. Walsh, Jeanette, 1944-
II. Beaton, Marilyn, 1947- III. Title.

RT6.N48M37 2008   610.7309718   C2008-906624-3

Cover Images:
Front Cover (left to right from upper left): Marcella French, Helen D. Penny,
Mary Galway, Ethel Williams, Gwen Thomas (left) with two of her classmates
in Wales, Jennie Wareham
Back Cover (top) Jennie Wareham in the dessert in Egypt, (bottom left)
Marcella French, N. Benson and M. Abbott in the Nursery of the Grace
Hospital, (bottom right) Alma Moores

The Canada Council | Le Conseil des Arts
   for the Arts | du Canada

We acknowledge the financial support of The Canada
Council for the Arts for our publishing activities.

We acknowledge the support of the Department of Tourism,
Culture and Recreation for our publishing activities.

Canadä

We acknowledge the financial support of the Government of
Canada through the Book Publishing Industry Development
Program (BPIDP) for our publishing activities.

Printed in Canada

Dedication

In memory of Baxter Marsh, and to all nurses of that era.

Contents

Introduction

For a young woman in Newfoundland in the 1920s or '30s there were few options when she considered her future. Outside of marrying and settling down to domestic life in the community, she could pursue secretarial work, teaching, or nursing. Of course most chose marriage and motherhood instead of following a career. For those who had a desire to care for the sick or who had an adventuresome spirit or who wished to travel, nursing offered the greatest opportunities. For some who lived in outport Newfoundland and Labrador, the adventure began when they left their small communities, often for the first time in their lives, and moved to St. John's to enter nursing school. Others used their nursing career as a springboard to new and sometimes exciting experiences after nursing school. As well, there were those who chose nursing after trying out a career in teaching or secretarial work.

In the mid 1980s, Marilyn Marsh interviewed 21 women who graduated from nursing between 1918 and 1949. Marilyn, also a nurse, had met these women in her career and felt they had a story to tell. These interviews, along with one completed by Joyce Nevitt in 1974 and given to Marilyn, provide a picture of what life was like for these women in those times. Due to health reasons, Marilyn was unable to complete the project and the interviews were stored away. In 2005, using grant money from the Association of Registered Nurses of Newfoundland and Labrador, the process of transcribing the interviews began, and with additional funding from the J. R. Smallwood Foundation, the transcriptions were completed in 2006. This project was considered research and subsequently the appropriate ethical approvals from the Human Investigation Committee at Memorial University were received. The tapes and transcribed interviews are to be stored at the Centre for Newfoundland Studies at Memorial University as a record of nursing in Newfoundland and Labrador and may be used as a source of data for future research purposes.

For our first book, *From the Voices of Nurses: An Oral History of Nursing in Newfoundland and Labrador*, we interviewed a group of 33 nurses. The majority of these women worked in nursing until the mid 1980s and gave us a 60-year picture of nursing in Newfoundland and Labrador. Through their recollections, the history of nursing education and practice in Newfoundland and Labrador, along with societal and historical influences impacting both, was captured for that era. This book, *A Life of Caring: 16 Newfoundland Nurses Tell Their Stories*, shares an earlier history of nursing through the personal stories of 16 women who practiced nursing primarily in the 1920s and '30s. At the time, the world was going through the Depression and the Second World War. The recollections of these women may not always be historically accurate, however, they are a reflection of their lived experiences and provide insight into who they were as women and nurses. Unlike the first book, these stories follow nurses outside the borders of the country of Newfoundland, and we get a glimpse at how they functioned and coped with their challenges.

The participants were interviewed in their homes. At the time of the interviews, the women ranged in age from 67 to 92 with an average age of 83. The length of each interview varied, with some requiring two visits to complete. The interview included information on each woman's family background, her nursing education and career in nursing. The questions elicited information on issues facing these nurses: the treatment of illnesses, available resources, the role of the nurse in the health care system of their day and the inevitable challenges they encountered in their practice. Not surprising, in the telling of their stories, the nurses also revealed information about socioeconomic conditions and historical events that impacted their work and lives. While initially shy talking about themselves, the participants became relaxed and enjoyed sharing their stories as the interview progressed. Talking about their nursing careers gave them an opportunity to appreciate their contributions to nursing and health care and to pass on valuable information about the evolution of the nursing profession to future generations of nurses.

Five interviews were excluded from this book because the participants' recollections of their nursing careers were limited. A sixth individual was excluded when a review of her records revealed she had left the school of nursing before completing her probationary period, although she had held herself out as a nurse all her life. She worked a number of years in health care settings but it is unknown in what capacity. This occurred at a time when there was no official nursing registry in Newfoundland and individuals could call themselves nurses without repercussion.

In Newfoundland, students were not admitted to nursing school as a class until the mid 1930s. Prior to then, they were admitted when a place became available at the hospital, and it was not unusual for one or two students to be admitted at varying times throughout the year. Subsequently, very few entered nursing directly from high school, and indeed most applicants to nursing were older. All but three were 21 or older. In this group, several of the participants opted for other careers before entering nursing. Three taught school for several years, one in Cartwright, Labrador. Two completed a business course, one of whom worked as assistant to two Newfoundland prime ministers, before choosing nursing. It became evident as the stories evolved that the majority came from families of "means" in that their fathers were local merchants or gainfully employed. This was not always the case for Newfoundland families in the 1920s and '30s.

All but one interviewee were from Newfoundland. Gwen Thomas graduated from nursing in South Wales and came to work as a district nurse in rural Newfoundland after the Second World War. Of those who studied in Newfoundland, all except Helen Penny graduated prior to 1939. This was at a time when the only schools of nursing that existed in Newfoundland were the St. John's General Hospital School of Nursing and the Grace General Hospital School of Nursing. Grace Hospital graduates completed the eighteen-month Maternity Program before returning to complete the RN Program. Five of the Newfoundland women interviewed traveled outside the province to study nursing.

In addition to recalling their nursing careers, the participants related stories of the social circumstances of the times and told of Newfoundland health agencies and health conditions long forgotten. Mary Galway told of her efforts to improve conditions for male patients at the Mental Hospital in the 1930s when their food was brought in buckets and served on tin plates. Cluda Grandy talked of her work with the travelling x-ray clinic on the Avalon Peninsula in an effort to eradicate tuberculosis. Marion Stone, one of the first industrial nurses in Newfoundland, shared stories of her work at the Imperial Tobacco Factory and her efforts to eradicate tuberculosis among the workers. From the interviews, we learn of Miss Whiteside, the Director for Public Health Nursing in Newfoundland in the 1930s, and her program to prepare nurses to work in rural Newfoundland. We learn of Cook Street, a home for unmarried mothers operated by the Salvation Army, and about Jensen Camp Hospital, the forerunner to the Sanatorium on Topsail Road. Within their stories, we hear of the poverty that existed in Newfoundland and the difficult conditions nurses experienced as they responded to the needs of their patients.

It is interesting to note these nurses' commitment to continuing education in areas like public health, midwifery, tuberculosis nursing, and x-ray therapy. Ethel Wells shares her experience doing an x-ray course following which she was expected to return to the Grace General Hospital to open the first x-ray department. Alma Moores and Eileen Shanahan tell about having to learn dentistry in preparation for their role as district nurses. From those nurses who worked in rural Newfoundland, we learn the magnitude of their workload, the conditions under which they worked, and their loneliness, but we also sense their independence, ingenuity, and commitment to their patients.

Some participants lived through two world wars. Three were directly involved in World War II. Gwen Thomas worked as a midwife in North London during the German bombings. Helen Penny served as an aerial photographer in the Royal Canadian Air Force while Jennie Wareham was a Nursing Sister in the South African Army and served in the North African desert from 1941 to 1945. Ethel Wells shares stories of working at the Sanatorium during that war. Surprisingly, the participants' stories reveal that many of the current issues facing nursing (e.g. quality of care, nursing shortages, and workload) are not new. On the one hand,

Mary Galway moved to New York to work because they were "screaming for nurses," while in Newfoundland, Marcella French tells us that "When we graduated, we didn't have a lot of expectations because there...weren't a lot of positions for graduates..." This was an era when nurses were invited to join the staff of a hospital, and positions for graduate nurses were limited because hospitals were primarily staffed by student nurses. Mary Feehan (whose interview is not included) related how she got employment: "We came on staff in 1939. You could scarcely buy a position on staff, but that year there was a flu epidemic and quite a few of the graduates at the General were off sick. Miss Mabel Smith applied to government to get a couple of nurses to fill in while the others were sick and that is how Miss Tobin and I got on staff at the General Hospital." A big issue in health care today is "wait times." Ethel Wells reveals that wait times for patients with tuberculosis were often detrimental to their illness: "They might be picked up early but by the time they got a bed they were much more advanced."

The nurses interviewed for this book were required to resign from their nursing position when they married. However, several of them provided nursing services within the community long after they were no longer employed in nursing. As one participant said, "The nurse was the only one there." Only those who never married continued in nursing. Their stories reveal the wide range of nursing experiences within the group, from private duty to nursing in general hospitals, public health, and cottage hospitals both in rural Newfoundland and South Africa, from working with tuberculosis patients in the sanatoriums of St. John's and Corner Brook, to working in nursing administration and education in Newfoundland and New York. As we compared the stories of participants educated in and outside of Newfoundland, it became clear that nursing education and practice in Newfoundland were not always as sophisticated as in other parts of the world, but their stories demonstrate the lengths that local agencies and nurses went to improve the care they provided to Newfoundlanders.

During the course of their careers, these nurses observed the impact of antibiotics on many illnesses and the introduction of therapies to treat tuberculosis, a disease once considered by many to be a death sentence. The participants practiced in an era when patients' recovery relied primarily on the nursing care they received. There was limited access to a broad range of medications, therapies and technology. Nurses working in rural Newfoundland were also faced with limited access to other professionals and relied on their own abilities and instincts. Within the hospital setting, all work related to patients passed through the hands of the nurse except that which fell within the physician's realm. The reality was that patients got better because of the nurse's ability to observe, make judgments, and intervene appropriately. For many, this reality provided them the most satisfaction, knowing it was their skills that helped the patient recover. Jennie Wareham: "I remember going off duty and worrying about a patient [with pneumonia]…then the next morning, the patient would be sitting up and his temperature normal. It was something to know it was only nursing care that kept them alive. It was very satisfying…" These women lived through a significant period of evolution in the practice of nursing.

The participants loved what they did and rarely expected any thanks in return. Helen Penny: "You didn't expect pats on the back as a nurse but sometimes you did get them from unexpected sources…" Many of them said they never thought of questioning the system or its expectations of them, they just did what had to be done. They took tremendous pride in what they did and set particularly high standards for themselves. Eileen Shanahan: "We knew that if we had any errors or mistakes or if there was any problem, it was mismanagement. I always had that in the back of my mind when I was in the district..." As they told their stories, these unassuming women had little appreciation for their vital contribution to improving the health of Newfoundlanders. In their view, they only did what was expected of them, and yet, it is amazing the lengths they went to care for their patients. While many of these nurses were not well known, each of them made a tremendous difference! They reflect the "silent majority" of nurses who care for their patients, try to make a difference in their practice, and expect little in return. As our predecessors, these nurses established the practice of nursing in Newfoundland and set out the expectations for the generations of nurses that followed them. As you read their stories you cannot but be proud of what they accomplished given the circumstances many of them faced and be motivated to continue their example.

CHAPTER 1:

Emma Parsons

"The big flu epidemic of 1920 was in the last year of my training. Students were the only ones on the ward to do anything. All the other nurses were home with the flu."

Emma Parsons was born in 1895 in Bay Roberts where her family was in business. She wanted to be a nurse from a very young age and while waiting for admission to nursing school taught in Cartwright, Labrador. Emma graduated from the Montreal General School of Nursing in 1920, where she received an award from the hospital board for her service during the 1920 flu epidemic.

"I had it in my mind to go nursing, but I took a teacher's training course and taught in two or three small schools while I was waiting for word to go to a hospital. Mr. Blackall, the General Superintendent of Education in St. John's, called and asked me to consider going to Labrador for the winter to teach. Mother wasn't pleased but I decided to go. That was 1914, the first year of the war.

"I had two days to get ready. We sailed on the last trip of the 'old' *Kyle* and it was very stormy. Cartwright was a small place with only about fifteen or twenty families. I taught there for a year and boarded with the clergyman, Reverend Kirby, and his family. The man in charge of the Hudson Bay was a Mr. Swaffly from England. He had three or four children who came to the school. The manager of the Hudson Bay Company was a man from Harbour Grace whom I knew. Cartwright was very good, but only the Hudson Bay Company employees had houses there. We had a nice little school near the church with twelve or fifteen students. We didn't have grades. We just taught reading, writing and arithmetic from primer up to the early teens. That was about all they did in school!

"In those days in Labrador, we had a boat connection in the summer and a dog team in the winter. We got mail a couple times during the winter, which they called overland mail. We didn't have fancy things, but we had everything we needed because the Hudson Bay Company was there. It was like a big store with everything in it, a trading post really and very busy. People came from all around. The Indians came to Cartwright by dog team from communities around Labrador to trade furs and get supplies. I never saw Indians in their communities because we weren't connected with them, so I didn't know anything about their living conditions.

"When I came back home, I didn't teach anywhere else until I went to the hospital. I don't know why I decided on Montreal. All I remember is putting in an application and waiting to get word. My parents didn't care because whatever we decided to do was all right with them as long as we got something to do. They saw that we got a good education and were ready to take a job.

"I went to Montreal by train. I didn't come home when I was in training because we never had money to travel and we didn't get holidays. We got very few days off while in training. After I graduated, I came home for Christmas every year. I always traveled by rail except one time when the boat came to pick up Earl Hague from Quebec. It took on some passengers and I came down to Newfoundland. That was the only time I came by boat.

"I don't know why I went into nursing. I had no special reason. There were quite a few Newfoundlanders in training in Montreal when I was there but I was the only one from Bay Roberts. My classmates were from all over Canada, with quite a few girls from the Maritimes and there were two or three Newfoundlanders in my class but they didn't finish. Several Newfoundlanders graduated the same time as I did.

"They gave us a list of stuff we needed when we went in training. Our probie uniform was ordinary blue, and after three or four months as a probie, our uniforms were made from a special material with MGH printed on it. We wore linen aprons with bibs that crossed over and fastened at the back and ordinary black shoes with rubber heels, which were quiet because you had to be quiet walking back and forth the wards. We made no noise on the ward!

"I remember the discipline. Nothing passed Miss Livingston! If we got word that we had to 'walk the red carpet' as we called it, we went with fear and trembling, I can tell you! She was likely to tell you to pack up and go! Her sister, Miss Gracie, was in the diet kitchen where we got our training for diabetes. She was VERY stern! Once I was blamed for something somebody else did. I was ready to pack and go home except the person who blamed me found out that she had blamed the wrong one.

"The Montreal General was a big hospital with mostly adult patients and we affiliated to other hospitals for maternity and pediatrics. We studied hard but we were never sure if we'd get through. We had no responsibility as far as the ward was concerned except if we did anything wrong. As probies we were taught to do things, and there were nurses on the ward who watched to see what we were doing. These were senior students in training and they told us the regular ward duties like bed making, washing bedpans, cleaning beds, cleaning bathrooms and everything. As probies we did a whole load of work! Some Head Nurses were strict and others weren't. Some were very helpful, but with others, you had to be on your p's and q's before you'd get any help. We went on duty every morning at seven o'clock, helped make the beds, and at nine o'clock we were in the classroom. Then we went back to the wards and worked from five to seven. Then we had our studies and other things to do.

"It was different from what it is today. We didn't have people on the wards like they do now. We did have doctors but nurses made all the beds and gave baths. Students didn't give any medication until the last year. We helped feed patients and got them out of bed if needed. We didn't do that very much though, because when patients were out of bed and could walk, they went home because there was always a waiting list for beds. If patients died, they were taken to a private room where we bathed them and the undertaker took them.

"Everything was so different. There was no insulin or anything like that. Most diseases were managed by diet. We had lots of patients with pneumonia who were treated with tepid sponge baths. The thing I remember most was the treatment for typhoid patients. We had a special ward for typhoid patients, but we only got a short training there. The patients had very high temperatures, and we'd put them in ice baths at a very low temperature for a few minutes to try to reduce their temperature. There was no other way of reducing it and so many of them died.

"The big flu epidemic of 1920 was in the last year of my training. The students were the only ones on the wards to do anything because all the nurses were home with the flu. I never got the flu first or last! I don't remember any nurse dying but they were too sick to come to work. In those days, when you got the flu, you never expected to come through, it was so bad! Only three or four of us stayed on duty and we did everything possible. Whatever the doctors ordered, like spongings to reduce the temperature, we did them. Patients with high temperatures got lots of fluids and that's about all they got. There was no penicillin, but we did have other kinds of drugs. The hospital was a big place and lots of patients came through but most died like flies. It was bad! We worked from early morning and sometimes it would be ten or eleven o'clock at night before we got off. A patient would die and before you got him ready for the morgue, somebody else was in the bed. You'd hardly get a chance to change the bed. There was such a waiting list to get in hospital, and if they didn't get treatment, they just died at home. That was all you could do; there was nobody to look after them! The flu was not just in Montreal; it was everywhere. A lot of people I knew in Cartwright died from the flu. There were only a couple of my friends left. People died like sheep! It was the worst kind of a flu you could have because pneumonia would set in. The Board of the Montreal General Hospital gave us a certificate for the work we did in the hospital during that flu epidemic.

"Residence was very friendly, but we were always on our p's and q's with the senior nurses. Everything was routine and you knew what to expect. We tried to do our best and not get in any trouble. But I enjoyed the nurses' residence. We had good times there. The residence was in the red light district of Montreal and there was always a crowd around in the night. It was a hard district and it was filthy, but the people were good to us because they knew us. It was only a five-minute walk from St. Catherine's down the old lane to the General, and whatever they did to other people, they never bothered us. They'd say, 'Here come the nurses,' or they'd take no notice of us at all. It didn't make any difference what hour of the night it was, we never had any trouble or ever had anything said to us. Two or three of us would go to shows, and I had two or three friends that I would visit. My best friend was a girl named MacIntosh and she lived outside Montreal; her father was a farmer. When we had our holidays, I used to visit them. They were great friends! I missed my parents, of course, but we were always in touch. We didn't get a chance to get out much and I don't remember any of the students having boyfriends. We could talk to male patients, but they weren't long conversations because we never had time. There were perhaps thirty or more beds in the ward and there wasn't time for conversation.

"We had very good meals, but it was the same food over and over again. We had two sittings for meals. We had a kitchen on the floor and we could always go there to get a glass of milk or make a cup of tea. When we were off duty we could go to the kitchen and get something to eat or go out to buy something or have something sent in. We always had a meal before we went to bed.

"After I graduated, I did special nursing in Montreal for five or six years. I never did any institutional work, except if I went to a hospital to do private duty with a patient. I had a room outside the hospital, and when I was off duty, I spent most of the time with two or three friends I had in Montreal.

"I came back to St. John's and did a few cases of private duty nursing off and on. I had a case where I'd go to give the patient's insulin every morning. I did that for nine years, every morning at nine o'clock, rain or shine. They'd come and shovel my driveway to get me out. Her daughter could give the needle, but the patient didn't want that. She wouldn't do it herself so I used to look after her. I also had two or three maternity cases. I never delivered any babies. Patients always had their own doctor to deliver the baby, but the nurse would be there with them. If there were anybody sick at home, like a senior, I'd go in and help them. I generally found something to do. Once, after I came home, I took a patient with a head injury to the Royal Victoria Hospital from the General Hospital because the mother couldn't go. She asked me to take him but he died up there.

"Nursing was a nice life for a time. I made good friends. I enjoyed my nursing training but our greatest worry was whether we'd get through."

CHAPTER 2:

Marion Stone

"The first thing I did [at the factory] was make all employees have a chest x-ray. We didn't employ anybody who didn't have a chest x-ray done. When I started that, they objected very strongly... but when I left in 1953, we had no employees with tuberculosis. I cleaned up tuberculosis at the company."

Marion Stone was born in Fogo where her father was a teacher. She graduated from the Boston City Hospital in 1926. In 1931, Miss Stone returned to Newfoundland to become one of its first industrial nurses, a position she held until her retirement in 1953. She provides some insight into the plight of workers as well as the social/living conditions in St. John's at the time. Miss Stone was interviewed by Joyce Nevitt in 1974.

"I don't know what took me to Boston, but I always had American leanings. My mother's people were there and I had a much-loved aunt in Boston. She suggested I come and I didn't need much pushing."

After graduation, Marion worked as a private duty nurse in

Boston for five years. "During the Depression in Boston, I registered to do everything but obstetrics. I hated obstetrics so much that I swore if I graduated I'd never touch it, and I never did. One day Central called me and said, 'Miss Stone, there is a case at Phillip's House.' I said, 'Not Phillip's House. I registered not to do obstetrics.' She said, 'Miss Stone, you're going to have to come down off your high horse. Do you know there's a Depression on?' I said, 'I know all about it, but I'm not going to do obstetrics.' And I never did, from the day I graduated! The operating room was my choice; I loved it! I worked in the OR at Boston City Hospital sometimes and I did a lot of work at the Peter Brent Brigham Hospital with Dr. Harvey Cushing. Of all the hospitals I worked at, the Brigham was my favourite. Everything was different. The nurses and doctors were different. Had I known about it, I would have liked to go in training there, but my people couldn't afford it. At the Brigham you had to pay for your tuition, uniforms, and books, whereas at Boston City Hospital we had to buy our uniforms and books. Our tuition was free and we got ten dollars a month in first year, twelve in second year, and fourteen in third year. It was a three-year training program. We lived in residence, a lovely home.

"I was lucky because it was during the Depression and hard to get a job, but my aunt was very well off and I didn't feel the Depression. She and I were closer than my mother and I. On my day off I'd visit her, and I never came back without a ten dollar bill. I think people in the United States felt the Depression more than any other part of the world. It was terrible! I had a case at the Belleview Hotel in Boston. She was a retired admiral's widow and lived there all her life after her husband died. We were looking out the window one day when a man came down from the next floor up. He jumped! I wouldn't say they felt the Depression too badly here in Newfoundland, but then Newfoundlanders have always been poverty stricken."

Marion Stone returned to Newfoundland in 1931, where she answered an advertisement in the newspaper for a job as industrial nurse at the Imperial Tobacco Company. "I applied and got it. It was an instant job. Things were in a primitive state when I went there, but I had the cooperation of management and we got things under control. When I went there first, one family had four cases of tuberculosis and was wiped out in a year. The first thing I did was to make all employees have a chest x-ray. We didn't employ anybody who didn't have a chest x-ray done. When I started it, they objected very strongly: 'We're not going.' I said, 'If you don't go, you won't have a job.' So they went. By the time I left there, they were coming to me: 'Nurse, can I go down for an x-ray?' When I left in 1953, we had no employees with tuberculosis. I cleaned up tuberculosis at the company."

The factory had 180 employees. Miss Stone's responsibilities varied from direct care of employees and their families to nutrition teaching and administrative duties. Much of her work focused on health education and illness prevention, an unusual approach for the time. "It was a grand place to work, a lovely company and the management was cooperative. I had a little office that was called the dispensary. It had a cot and all the equipment necessary. My caseload varied, from minor problems such as dysmenorrhea, colds, cuts, and bruises to more major problems such as heart attacks and epilepsy. We didn't have any maternity cases because we didn't employ married women. Once they got married, they left. Sometimes they tried to put one over on me, but they went anyway. That was the rule in the company and they knew it. I saw all staff who were sick. They reported in between 9 and 10 a.m., and I visited older patients in their homes in an advisory capacity and sent for the doctor if necessary.

"I started rounds at ten o' clock. In one department, there was a vat on the floor with boiling water and bread soda in it. The trays where the beaver tobacco was made were washed off in this vat. One day somebody carelessly left the guard off the vat and a man fell in. I had to fish him out. He had on Stanfield woolen underwear which had gone into his flesh. I had him rushed to the hospital immediately. He lived but was in hospital for a long time. In cases like that they got workmen's compensation. We also had group life insurance which I looked after. We had a cafeteria which was under my supervision and I taught nutrition and health. The company was really far advanced for its time.

"When I got the job, Mr. Patterson said to me, 'Miss Stone, you're entitled to your breakfast and lunch.' I went to get a cup of tea, and when I took the sugar can out of the cupboard, five hundred and fifty-five million cockroaches came out! Mr. Patterson said, 'You'll get used to that, Miss Stone,' and I said, 'I never will!' We got the exterminator in but we never did get rid of them. They'd be gone during the day, but if you turned the light on at night they were still there. Going home that first afternoon after work, my father was waiting for me at the railway station. When we were on the streetcar, he said, 'How did you like the job?' I said, 'Father, I don't want to hear one thing about that job!' I was so mad! I think Mr. Patterson had me sized up because he said, 'Miss Stone, what we'll do is let things run for a year and if at the end of the year we don't like you, we'll tell you, and if you don't like us, you tell us.' I said, 'You go fly a kite. I'll be gone out of here before Christmas.' But things got worse in the States with the Depression…there was no work. So I stayed put because I had a very good salary."

In the early 1930s, the Imperial Tobacco Company closed temporarily. "That was for political reasons. They had a riot at the Colonial Building. Sir Richard Squires was premier [prime minister] at the time but they cleared him out and Alderdice got in as premier [prime minister]. He was also the chief director of the Imperial Tobacco Company and thought to be in conflict of interest. To prove that he had no conflict of interest, he closed the company. All the employees were put out of work, but people got a closing payment. After the factory closed, Mr. Patterson sent me around to visit all the homes, to see what they were getting. I found that some were only getting two or three dollars a month. When they were working and got sick, the factory paid them, but all they got from the government was six cents a day. Here's a list of the amounts of relief they received, dated January 22, 1932: a family of thirteen got $4.50 a month; another with seven in the family got $2.00 relief; one family of eight got $4.00; while a family of six got $4.00; and another family of six got $3.50. That's all they got for welfare and the factory paid them nothing. Many didn't survive! They died of pneumonia and tuberculosis. Eventually they brought all the foremen back to do painting, scrubbing, and cleaning, just to give them something to do, but they only went in to work in the mornings and had a whale of a time.

"It's no good to tell you about St. John's then. People lived in shambles, shacks! If there was a death in the family, there was no place to wake them because there were no funeral parlours. They waked them in the kitchen beside the kitchen stove. They had to bury people very quickly! I remember one girl who had pneumonia. There was only a kitchen, bedroom, and another room in the house, and I don't know how many were in the family. The weather was very bad that winter and the house was snowed in on the side where the window was. There was no air of any sort. I called the doctor and Dr. Henderson came up. The first thing he did was put his foot through the window and kicked it out. Telling about it now seems impossible but that's what went on then. The people knew how to survive; they'd been doing it a long time.

"I haven't nursed since 1953. I came home in 1931 and worked at the Imperial Tobacco Company until it closed up in 1953, twenty-two years."

CHAPTER 3:

Ethel Wells

"The program wasn't for nurses...but I was to come back and open the x-ray department. In the last lecture I felt like crying because I didn't think I knew anything. They'd say, 'Miss Wells, if there's anything you don't know or understand, just let us know.' I didn't know what I knew and what I didn't know!"

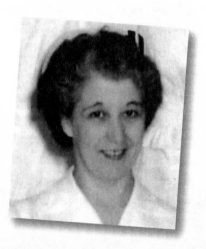

Ethel Wells was born in 1899 in Bonavista. Following a brief career in teaching, she completed the Maternity Nursing Program at the Grace Hospital in Halifax in 1924 and the Diploma

Nursing Program at the Grace Hospital in Windsor, Ontario, in 1928. Following completion of an x-ray course in Chicago, Miss Wells opened the first x-ray department at the Grace Hospital in St. John's. She retired as Matron of the Sanatorium in 1959 after 25 years.

"I began teaching in a one-room Salvation Army School in Charleston around 1917. After school, I went to young people's meetings and got interested in the Salvation Army. Soon I was leading the meetings. I joined the Army, although my father got in trouble with the United Church clergymen because he let me go to the Army and not to church on Sundays.

"I taught for about four or five years in several one-room schools in places like Hopeall, Trinity Bay, and Seal Cove, Fortune Bay. The last school year I taught was in Bonavista because I was going into officer training at the Army College, but when they did my medical they discovered I had TB so I landed in the Sanatorium as a patient! That ended my teaching. I think I got TB when I was teaching at Seal Cove because I looked after a Salvation Army officer whose father was the merchant. She was in the Sanatorium for two years and came home to die. I stayed with her every second night. I taught school during the day and stayed with her at night. I had one night in bed and one night napping in a chair. I used to hold her in my arms facing me. I didn't know anything about nursing then!

"These places were very isolated and there was only the teacher and a Salvation Army officer, so you were a bit of everything. Oh, the queer things that happened! If a couple had a squabble they'd send for whichever one was home. I had a little child who sat in a boiler of soup just taken off the stove. My brother worked in a store and some agent had given him samples of Zambuk. He had given me a pocket full of these samples and that's what I used to treat the child. You never saw better healing because all his skin had been left in the pot!

"We had a woman who was hemorrhaging. I didn't know at the time but she must have been aborting because that's where she was bleeding from. The officer with me was as young as I was, but she had a bit more experience and insight into things because she had been in officer training whereas I came straight from home. We took turns putting her legs up and her head down to elevate the bleeding part, and the bleeding stopped. I don't know if she would have died or not, but we probably saved her life. She did abort but I didn't know anything about abortions. I didn't know anything about childbirth! I suppose we knew what was happening, but in those days we didn't see and hear about it on television. The only news we got was written in the post office in Bonavista.

"Sometime in 1919, I went to the Sanatorium and was in bed six months with a temperature. About a year later, I started to work on the wards; Dr. Rendell got staff by recruiting from the patients. If you showed any sign of being good you got a job. Just as I started to work at the Sanatorium they moved the men from Jensen Camp, which was a hospital built for soldiers returning from overseas. The soldiers went there first when they came back to be weeded out, and a lot of them had TB. They were moved to the Sanatorium on Topsail Road where two long wards with about 70 beds on each ward had been built. They were the largest wards ever! There were three rows of beds: one on each side, one in the middle, and the nurses' station in the centre.

"After I left the San, I took a job at Jensen Camp as a school-teacher. Some local ladies asked the Salvation Army if they would use the country home there to help the street girls. I guess you would call them prostitutes. The Army tried it for a year with the understanding that they could stop whenever they liked. The officer I was with at Seal Cove was appointed by the Army to be in charge of these girls. We lasted about nine months, but it was quite a problem because they were a pretty tough crowd. There were fifteen of them. First they'd pull the phone receiver off the wall so you were at their mercy, then they'd use anything to attack you. While we were there, they did fine, but after we left, a graduate nurse and teacher went to look after the place. They lasted three weeks before they ended up at the General Hospital, pretty badly beaten up. The nurse had her head split open in several places. The local ladies worked hard but they gave it up.

"They were calling for nurses during the First World War, and I remember being in church one Sunday night and crying through the service because I wasn't old enough to be a nurse. I thought I only had to say I wanted to go into nursing, put my hat and coat on, and go. I don't know if that started me thinking about nursing because I had always had a leaning that way anyway. If anybody was sick in the community I liked to look after them. I did a lot of that. I loved looking after older people. In 1922, after I left Jensen Camp, the Army sent me to the Grace in Halifax to do the maternity and gynecology program. I graduated in 1924 but was a bit late finishing because I had two months sick time and had to work that in after graduation. We had the usual lectures in maternity and gynecology, which were taught by doctors except for the nursing part. Our teachers were trained Army officers. It was an excellent training program and I wouldn't have missed it for anything.

"We did some deliveries ourselves but not at the Grace because it was a university training school for doctors and they did deliveries. The first thing we did when a patient came in was phone the doctor, then phone the university to get the students on call. I assisted with numerous caesarean sections. Once we were trained to run a case, the nurse gave the anesthetic. I often wonder how we did it because we weren't trained to give anesthetics for caesarean sections. We'd put them under with a little chloroform and keep them under with ether. For an ordinary or late forceps delivery, it was a light anesthetic, and for a long labour or a high forceps delivery, a deep anesthetic was given. The baby would have bruises, but I only saw a baby affected once. The father was a doctor and refused permission for a caesarean. The doctor doing the delivery didn't want to use forceps because he knew it was going to be a hard job. The baby's neck broke! All you could see was the flesh on the baby's neck stretch out. That was the worst thing I ever saw! I was giving the anesthetic even with two doctors in the room. The husband just watched and said, 'I guess you were right, weren't you?' There was never any sign of life so we never knew if the baby was dead before the neck was broken. It was never questioned but that's what happened. There were some hard maternity cases!

"At the Grace in Halifax they liked my accent because I think people from Bonavista talk a bit like the Irish. Each morning we got our assignments and that evening we'd give the Head Nurse a report. She'd repeat everything I was told to do that morning and I'd say I did it. This went on every evening and finally I asked to see Matron. I told her what was going on and said, 'Major Clarke, I work as well or better than most of the nurses here and what I do, I do well.' She laughed and said, 'Miss Wells, don't mind them. They only want to hear you say, "Sure now, I'm after doing that."' They loved hearing it! But I didn't know; it took me a while to catch on! I stopped saying it, and even now I still squirm if I hear myself say it.

"We had more septicemia then because there were no antibiotics. When I was a probie, I looked after a patient with septicemia. It was a problem for the training school because the patient, her husband, and the doctor only wanted me to look after her and she was so sick. They taught me how to scrub before

I handled her and what to do when I left her. I wore a gown, gloves, and mask, and scrubbed so much I was sore. I had to do it because the doctor was watching and I could have gotten septicemia. I scrubbed too well for any bug to live! I had a similar experience with a doctor who was a maternity and gynecology professor at Dalhousie and wanted me to care for his wife. His wife said later, 'I bet they didn't tell you at the hospital that we asked for you, did they?' The school didn't like putting nurses in training on with patients.

"I returned to the Grace in St. John's as a maternity staff nurse before I went into the first diploma class at the Grace School in Windsor, Ontario. I got one year credit for the maternity program, so it took me three and a half years to train as a graduate nurse. I never saw a tonsillectomy until I went to Windsor and that was one of the first things I wanted to see. In Windsor I lived in residence for the first time. It was a new building just opened. The hospital had a cottage for our weekends and days off, but we had to get to that by rowboat. That was so pleasant. I enjoyed every bit of it.

"When I graduated from Windsor, I came back when the new Grace Hospital opened in St. John's. We were perhaps the first three graduate nurses at the hospital and we worked pretty long hours, 15 and 16 hours most of the time. I worked up to 24 to 48 hours without getting time off, because when babies came, they came like caplin in schools! But that was seldom. You might get an hour of sleep, then had to get up! There was a Miss A. who never got up for anything. She'd toggle around to see if everything was all right. She was more of a hindrance!

"Doctors came in for emergencies at the Grace but not for Cook Street, which was a place for unmarried mothers. A graduate nurse who was an Army officer was in charge. We went there to deliver babies; it was part of our day. Occasionally the doctor would send them to the Grace to be delivered if things weren't going well. As soon as an unmarried mother landed in the hospital, Miss A. would put a ring on her finger and she would be called Mrs. So and So until she was discharged. Nobody in the hospital knew who they were except the nurse who was on when they came in. The patient would be put on a ward and wouldn't be treated differently, but these girls spent a lot of time waiting for their babies to be adopted. It took a lot of time out of their lives.

"I went to Chicago from the Grace to learn how to do x-rays and electrotherapy. The program wasn't for nurses but the hospital sent me to come back and open their x-ray department. In the last lecture I felt like crying because I didn't think I knew anything. They'd say, 'Miss Wells, if there's anything you don't know or understand, let us know.' I didn't know what I knew or didn't know! I could have swamped them with questions. We had no books, only techniques; there was no help to refer to! They demonstrated how to do the different x-rays and you had to remember everything they told you! It was a big hospital with seven or eight hundred patients and we practiced on them. We watched the patients and gave them so much time and so much dosage. That was the pioneer days of x-rays! They figure I am the only one who worked with x-rays in the early days and didn't get x-ray burns. You didn't wear protective clothing or gloves. They didn't know anything about protection!

"I also learned electrotherapy in Chicago. There were seven different machines; one was called diathermy, another called autocompensation, and the ultraviolet machine, which was very successful for skin conditions because most were caused by an allergy, although allergies weren't thought about in 1928. I had a patient whose hands were raw, red, burning and itchy. He suffered with it for years and one day some doctor came along and said, 'I don't suppose you're allergic to rubber?' He couldn't use anything with rubber like overshoes or a raincoat, not even a pencil with an eraser.

"One of the electrotherapy treatments I learned in Chicago was a wave machine where you picked up the motor points. I only remember the popliteal motor point, which I used when patients were in casts, and you felt the popliteal because you couldn't see it with the cast on. When you used the machine with the cast off, you could see the muscle contracting. It worked like a physiotherapist would, relaxing and contracting the muscle. You didn't worry when the cast came off because the patient's muscles were in good form and they were able to walk. It was time consuming because the operator had to stay with the machine, but I managed to get through all the appointments each day. There was no physiotherapy and we used these machines until the first physiotherapist came here.

"These machines were at the Grace when I came back. I made a few faux pas in the beginning. Sometimes, when you dusted, you'd break the connections. One day I couldn't get any power in the x-ray machine so I called the service man. He came, looked around and pulled down a button I had pushed up. He gave me a look and left! I felt so foolish! After that, the first thing I looked at was that button. The General had an x-ray machine a year before us but we never got together. St. Clare's got their x-ray machine a year after us, and by that time I was really established and able to work on my own. They'd get in touch with me and I'd go over and help them out. We had a good liaison. The only thing I recognize now is the x-ray table and it is as hard as ever. I had a scan done and refused to lay on my tummy on the hard table. I said, 'If you use a bit of sponge rubber, the x-ray will go through it.' They used it and it turned out fine.

"In 1935, I went to the Sanatorium as Director of Nursing and was there until I retired in 1959, about 25 years. You had to retire at age 60 then. Some of the greatest changes in my career were in tuberculosis treatment. At first bed rest was the big treatment, along with lots of fresh air. Cold, fresh air! The nurses and patients had to dress up because they spent a lot of time outdoors. Government provided nurses with a cape, sweaters, and gloves because they had to make beds outdoors. There was no heat except in the bathroom. When I was a patient there, we congregated in the bathroom to warm our hands, but the nurse would bundle us out. When I went there to work in '35, there was still no heat on the wards, only lots of fresh air. If we closed a window, the patients would have a fit.

"We had problems giving the TB drugs when they first came in because a lot of the staff became allergic to them. We didn't get many patients with an early lesion because they might be picked up early, but by the time they got a bed they were so advanced most patients needed to have a pneumothorax done. One of the first surgical procedures to treat TB was a phrenicotomy, which was done to remove or destroy the phrenic nerve, but everybody who had it done got very distressed with stomach symptoms which were attributed to the phrenic nerve. Then they started to crush the phrenic nerve, and this was done for years, even after thoracoplasty was started. We sent Dr. Jasmin away and he came back as the first permanent staff surgeon at the Sanatorium. He did full or partial thoracic lobectomies for many years.

"I was at the Sanatorium during the Second World War. Having to cover 500 windows every night during the blackout was a big problem. Some of the patients were devilish, and would take off the blackout covering. Then we'd get calls from the Goulds Road telling us that lights were showing. They'd say, 'In the northwest corner on the south side,' and I'd have to try and find it. At first, I didn't know what they were talking about, but before the war was over I knew more about it. We had to have nurses on duty all the time doing ARP [Air Raid Protection] duty every night. They'd check but they still had their jobs to do.

"I enjoyed everything! I loved my training and hated for it to be over. I kept in touch with my classmates in the beginning, and several of them came to work at the Grace in St. John's because the Army shifted their people around frequently. But I didn't keep up any correspondence because when I came back to the Grace I hardly had time to write to those who belonged to me."

After retirement from the Sanatorium, Miss Wells continued to work in nursing for another 12 years, primarily doing private duty, and she finally retired from nursing in 1972.

CHAPTER 4:

Alma Moores

"I did a good many deliveries at Cook Street. Sometimes the doctor would come, but other times the doctor would ring and say, 'If the baby is coming, you go ahead and let me know.' I was never taught how to do deliveries. I just watched what they were doing and learned on the job."

Alma Moores Mullins was born in Bay Roberts. Before entering nursing, she taught for a brief time. Alma graduated from the Grace Hospital Maternity Program in 1926 and returned there to complete the Diploma Program in 1931. She worked briefly with public health in St. John's before moving to Rencontre as District Nurse. Although Alma 'gave up' nursing after she married, she continued to care for the people of Rencontre and surrounding communities.

"I left teaching for nursing because I wanted to be a nurse. I was 19 when I applied to the Grace Hospital. My sister was in charge of the Salvation Army cadets on Springdale Street, but rather than go there as a cadet, I went to the hospital. Brigadier

Fagner had a meeting and when the women saw me, they said, 'You're too young to go in training. You'll have to wait another year.' I was sent to Cook Street, a home run by the Salvation Army where unmarried mothers had their babies. I mainly looked after the children, but I also did a good many deliveries. Sometimes the doctor would come, but other times the doctor would ring and say, 'If the baby is coming, you go ahead and let me know.' I was never taught how to do deliveries! I just watched what they did and learned on the job. It wasn't until I was in the caseroom at the Grace that I saw everything. While I was at Cook Street I went to the Grace five times a week for lectures. Sometimes someone, maybe one of the doctors, would take me to the hospital because it was a long walk. I stayed at Cook Street until November 1924, and then went to the Grace.

"Just before Christmas of that year I got sick with typhoid fever! I was working in the nursery and when it came time for dinner, I said to Miss Ensign, 'I'm not going to dinner. My throat is too sore.' She said, 'You go off duty at 3:30 and come back at 5:30.' I said, 'I won't be coming back because I'm going to bed.' I was sick! They didn't send me to the Fever Hospital and I always wondered why. My mother came to stay with me for six weeks. We were in the basement at the Grace. They moved all the nurses and left me in the room alone and kept another bed there for Mom.

"The Grace had an eighteen-month maternity training program then. We didn't have many patients because there was only the first floor. There was a big room for twelve married women who had babies. We called it 'down in the basement.' When I was on night duty, I had to look after them and the patients upstairs. Some mothers would be in bed fourteen days and wouldn't get up until the tenth day. They couldn't sit up and the nurses looked after them. I think a lot of these women were very tired and glad to be in hospital to get a rest. They worked pretty hard at home. In those days they got six dollars a month dole from government. It wasn't very much!

"I graduated in 1926 and worked at the Grace until 1929. Then the Grace became a general hospital and we had to go back to school to become graduate nurses. It took another 18 months after we finished the maternity program. Eleven of us graduated in 1931 and I was the first graduate nurse from the Grace General. As students, we wore a blue dress with a white bib and cuffs just below the elbow, which we washed ourselves. We wore black shoes and stockings, but after graduation we wore white shoes and stockings.

"In first year we didn't get a cent, but after that, we got $2.79 every Friday. The first time I got mine, I put the money underneath my mattress, because I didn't know where else to put it. We were going out for ice cream when we got off at 7 p.m., and when I went to get my money, it was gone! I told Brigadier Fagner and she said, 'They lost a lot of money today.' I had to wait until the next Friday to get any money. After that, I put it in my trunk.

"There were only a few doctors at the Grace then, Drs. Roberts, Moores, McPherson, Black, Blunt, Carnell and Greaves, and most of our lectures were given by the doctors. Nurses gave lectures in between. When we did maternity, nurses came up from the General Hospital and stayed for two months and we had classes together. Whatever nurse was on duty taught the maternity classes and looked after patients.

"When they opened the Grace General, it had a second floor. We had lots of room and lots of operations. There were two rooms, one for tonsils and little things and the other was for big operations like appendix or gallbladders. Ada Gillard and I were the only two nurses in the operating room. We'd start at 8:00 a.m. to get the operating room ready for the doctors. We had to get gowns and gloves ready and set up surgical trays with scalpels. Then we had to dress for the operation. The doctor put them to sleep with chloroform and ether. An appendix operation would be done at 8:00 or 9:00 a.m., and the patient would be there all day. One of the nurses from the ward would come down to sit with the patient until they were ready to go back. After the operation two of us did all the sterilizing and cleaned everything in the room. We didn't have girls to wash blood from the linen before sending it to the laundry. We had to do everything! I worked there for eight months then got sick. I couldn't go back to the operating room so Brigadier Fagner put in Violet Best, who was in our class. She also had to look after the maternity part and we were still students! I looked after the caseroom, and if anybody came to have their babies when I was on night duty, I'd phone the doctor. He'd say, 'Is everything all right? Well, go ahead and deliver the baby, then phone and let me know how things are.' I had to do that a good many times!

"After graduation the Salvation Army sent me back in charge of Cook Street. I wore a white uniform because I was the supervisor. I was there a month when they transferred me to the Halifax Maternity, and I stayed there for three or four years. I was a captain then and got $5.75 every Friday. I came home to Bay Roberts and went to Ottawa to see my sister on that money. I also visited another sister in London, Ontario, and went to Montreal before I came back to St. John's.

"Things happened with patients in Halifax that I really don't want to talk about. They were sad. If a patient was in labour, three or four interns from Dalhousie would come to see what was going on. There was one couple, a very tall man with a tiny wife. She was in labour and came to the Halifax Grace. She finally had her baby but it died. She got pregnant again and everything went all right, but the first time…things happened.

"When I first went into training, I'd get a pain in my back and chest every once in a while. It would pass off but I'd be in bed for a couple of days. Dr. Roberts would say, 'One of these days we'll have to operate on you.' In Halifax I got the same pain three or four times, and Drs. McDonald and Morton (from Brigus) operated and discovered I had an ulcer. I came home on a diet and six months rest. I lost a lot of weight.

"I didn't go back to Halifax but stayed here to work at the Grace. I left there to work with Miss Whiteside on Duckworth Street for a year. She was in charge of the government nurses. We went on duty at 8:00 a.m., and if anybody were having a baby two of us would go to different areas of the city. We'd do the delivery and look after them. Dr. Power, a dentist, used to take out teeth three times a week and I'd assist him. One day, I'd inject the cocaine and he'd take the teeth out. The next day, he'd inject it and I'd pull the teeth. I did that for a year. I'd say, 'What am I going to do if I'm ever sent to an outport?' and he'd say, 'You'll be better than I am. If you're sent anywhere and somebody has a toothache, they can always come to you.'

"Miss Whiteside sent me in charge of Argentia hospital. The doctor there would say every morning, 'Perhaps I'll operate today,' and he'd do it after supper or in the night. Several times I said to him, 'This is not right. I don't have any time off,' because whenever he did an operation we had to stay on duty. I stayed a year anyway and Miss Whiteside sent me to Rencontre, Fortune Bay. That was 1940 and I stayed there for two years before I came home.

"You could only get to Rencontre by boat, and my area was Stone's Cove, Hare Harbour, Anderson's Cove, Tickle Beach, Bay de Norde, Pool's Cove and Turnip Cove. Every day I'd get a message to go, and the fishermen would take me to the different places or someone came for me. I would just be back in Rencontre from Stone's Cove or another place and have to go to Pool's Cove. Things were pretty hard in Rencontre. People were getting six dollars a month dole but they weren't as poor as some other areas. Only about five men got cheques, and most of them were working with the fisheries department.

"There were two stores in Rencontre, the Coffin's and Keeping's. My surgery was across from Coffin's and I'd go up there every day. The people paid five dollars a year to Mr. Smith at Harbour Breton to cover whatever medical help they needed. He visited the different places around Fortune Bay by boat and collected the money.

"I got fifty dollars a month while I was nursing in Rencontre. One of the nurses told me that if anybody gave me money, I should keep it. But if I delivered a baby and they paid me, I gave the money to Mr. Smith. But lots didn't! My father died while I was there, but I couldn't get back because the telegram came a few minutes after the steamer left. It was winter and a lot of snow. It would have taken three or four days to come on the train.

"I fell in love in Rencontre. I got married in Bay Roberts, went back to Rencontre, and lived there for 25 years. I 'gave up' nursing after I married, but they always came to me because I was the only nurse. Then Dr. Miller asked me to stay on after I got married, so I'd go up to the surgery two or three times a week or if anybody got sick. I'd give them pills but we only had aspirin and cod oil. It was five cents for aspirin and twenty-five cents for a big bottle of cod oil. You didn't have much to offer in the way of pain medicines, just aspirin! There was a very sick man in Stone's Cove and his son came for me in a boat. It was a real stormy day and one of the fishery department boats said they'd take me over. My husband came with me and as we went out to sea the waves came in. Oh my, we had some job getting there! We landed and another boat came for me. Eventually I got there. I was sent to Harbour Breton because Dr. Paton went on his honeymoon and I had to replace him for two weeks. I went back and forth to the women who were having babies. I'd live with them and go back to the hospital after they delivered. If they wanted anything, they'd phone or somebody would come to get me and I'd go back.

"My husband worked with the fisheries department looking after the caribou, moose, trout and salmon. He went from Marystown to Port aux Basques by boat, and I made seventeen trips with him. Then the department said only employees could go on the boat. So I'd go on the steamer and meet my husband in places like Gaultois, St. Alban's, or Milltown. Sometime in the 1960s we went to Belleoram and I was walking with my daughter who taught there. Three or four people came up and asked if I'd go to their houses because somebody was sick. I went up to see how they were and to tell them what to take because there was no doctor there. Another two men went to the boat I came on and asked if I was aboard because a woman had her baby but no afterbirth came. They wanted to know if I would go. I went but there was no water to wash, so I got hold of the placenta and did what I could. I found out later that these men had gone 20 miles to St. Alban's for the doctor, but he wouldn't come. He said, 'Send her to Harbour Breton.' Sometimes people were sent to Harbour Breton but rarely. The men got back from St. Alban's just as I arrived, so they came to see what I could do. Afterwards the woman sent me a lovely cushion."

In 1962, Mrs. Mullins spent eleven months in hospital recovering from surgery to remove a brain tumour. During that time, her husband died, but she didn't know until she recovered. She was discharged from hospital on June 3, 1963, and almost 24 years to the day, on June 1, 1987, she participated in this interview. Clearly, Mrs. Mullins' recollections of her nursing career were not impacted by her illness. Neither was her opinion of her career. When asked about her choice of nursing, she responded, "If I had to live my life over, perhaps I would have gone into nursing. I did have a variety of nursing experiences."

CHAPTER 5:

Lillabelle Oke

*"…the chief teacher used to call out, 'One bright and
shining light wrote…' then she'd call out our mistakes. One day
we were talking about specialized hospitals and it was my
turn. She said 'It's not much good asking you. You wouldn't know,
coming from the sticks.'"*

When Lillabelle Oke applied to nursing school, she was told she
was too young. The director advised her to "go out and have a life
because nursing is hard work." Following completion of a business
course, Miss Oke worked for two Newfoundland prime ministers
before entering nursing school at St. John's Hospital in Brooklyn,
New York. After graduation, she worked as Head Nurse at Childs
Hospital in Albany, New York, with disabled children each
summer in Saratoga, and finally, as School Nurse at St. Agnes
School in New York.

"When I finished at Spencer, I went to see Miss Taylor to
apply for nursing school, but she said I was too young and she

couldn't take me. She suggested I go out and have a little bit of life first. I took a business course at Mercy Convent and went to work in Dr. Blackall's office for six weeks.

"I went to work at Baine Johnson's store and left there to be married, but the marriage fell through and I had nothing to do. My friend was leaving the prime minister's office and I thought working there would be interesting. I felt sure I would be hired if I spoke to Mr. Monroe, the prime minister. He told me to come to his door at seven o'clock the next evening. I went and he said, 'Lillabelle, I shouldn't have had you come because the job is yours. Your friends at Baine Johnson highly recommended you.'

"In the meantime, I visited an aunt in New York. She was on the board of St. John's Hospital in Brooklyn and told the Director of Nurses that I was always going to be a nurse. The Director of Nurses said, 'Lillabelle, if you ever decide to go in nursing, don't hesitate because you won't need an interview here.'

"I had been working with the prime minister, Sir Richard Squires, for four years, but my father wasn't happy because I was working a lot of nights. One day he said, 'If you're still hipped on nursing, how about it?' I wrote to St. John's Hospital, got my papers, and went to Baine Johnson because they wanted a businessman's reference. I told Sir Richard when I was set to go a month later! I went in January 1929 and graduated in 1932 at age 29. I loved every minute of it! I thought I'd be with kids just out of school, but there were seven older girls who had done other things. Emma Mifflin, my friend, went with me and we loved it.

"Thirty-two nurses graduated that year with three Newfoundlanders: Emma Louise Mifflin, Myrtle Hefferton and myself. Four prizes were awarded: one each for Best All Around Medical, Best All Around Surgical, Best All Around Obstetrical, and Best All Around Nurse. I received the Best All Around Medical Nurse, and Hefferton won Best All Around Nurse

"Our chief teacher was a German woman, Miss Heiner, who was a bit sarcastic. She'd say, 'One bright and shining light wrote…' then she'd call out our mistakes. One day we were talking about specialized hospitals and it was my turn to speak, and she said, 'It's not much good asking you. You wouldn't know, coming from the sticks.' I answered, 'Would you be looking for Brooklyn Eyes, Ears and Throat?' And she said, 'I guess you do know.' She was something!

"We helped each other because we could not go to the wards until we were perfect in the classroom. One day in class, Miss Heiner said, 'Miss Oke, pay attention to your own book instead of somebody else's.' I saw her after class and said, 'I'm sorry, Miss Heiner, but I have to tell you I didn't like your remark. I take your notes in shorthand, type them, and then my book goes around the class.' She said, 'Oh, you'll be able to help me!' After that, I used to do odd things for her.

"I was told to check on Mr. So and So's bed bath. We washed the face, hands, chest, back, and legs, then put the feet in the basin. I washed the patient's chest, back, face, and hands. All I could think about was asking him to finish his bath because if he couldn't do it, we got the orderly to finish the bath. I soaped up the cloth, gave it to the patient, and said, 'Would you mind finishing your bath?' Outside the curtain, the supervisor who was checking said, 'Miss Oke, you can't be passed on that bath. If you look behind the curtain, the patient is washing his feet.' He didn't know what else was left!

"The Episcopalian Sisters in the hospital would come to say prayers each morning and evening and we were reported if we didn't go. We were told that whatever happened or whatever we were doing, we were supposed to go to prayers. We were each assigned four or five patients who had to be done before we got a break, so if you were doing patients, it was hard to leave for prayers. One morning, just as Sister Theresa started to say the prayers, Marion Horwood, who was a practical nurse and from Newfoundland, came in with a bedpan and put it down in front of Sister and said, 'We were told that no matter what we were doing, we had to go to prayers!' So she came to prayers! She was practical all right!

"At Christmas, we exchanged gifts. Everyone's name went in the box regardless of who they were in the hospital. I would always get a teapot or a tea set with a package of teabags – something related to me and my tea! Anyway, whose name should I draw but Miss Heiner! I bought a flashlight and wrapped it up with a little verse.

> *'Oh the bright and shining lights come from far and near.*
> *Some are dark and some are fair.*
> *When Miss Heiner is finished, we know quite a lot.*
> *And we enjoyed very much our life in the spot.'*

"She asked one of the interns, 'Do you know who had my name?' and he said, 'No.' She said, 'I wish I could find out.' But she never did!

"I never did anything but I wasn't caught. We took a skeleton up on the roof one day and took his picture! Who should get on the elevator as we were coming down but Miss Heiner! She said, 'I hope you haven't hurt him. Take him back to the classroom! You're not the first class that's done this.' She was really good, you know!

"My sister had graduated from the same hospital. After she married she'd bring over the baby and some cookies and we'd have afternoon tea in my room. One day there was a knock on the door and I said, 'Come in if you're good looking.' In walked Miss Heiner. 'I'm not good looking but you have to go down to the prenatal clinic because so-and-so took ill suddenly.' I went to the clinic and they helped me as much as they could. I was first in my class to go on night duty and to the operating room, the first to do it all!

"On the maternity floor we washed patients before supper and took their temperatures. One night as I was handing out basins, this woman said to me, 'Never mind, Miss Oke, me darling. Why would you be going through the trouble of giving me the soakin? I could have washed at the spit.' I said, 'How did you know I was Miss Oke?' and she said, 'Sure, you were here last year and the year before that. This is my third year in.' I said, 'That must have been my sister.' She said, 'Well you talk like her.' I said, 'Of course, we both come from Newfoundland. Where do you come from?' and she said, 'St. Mary's Bay, Newfoundland.' She was living in the States and this was her third baby in three years. She was as Irish as could be! She meant she could have washed at the faucet.

"Dressings were not changed every day unless the patient was in a private room, and it depended on how much drainage. The incisions were cleaned with Lysol. On Sundays you straightened the linen closet, cleaned the utility room, and scoured everything in the place. We used to say we were God's gift to them! The poor probies couldn't do a lot of things but we could do that. Nursing was work but I still enjoyed it. I didn't mind work because my father was sick for a long time before I went in nursing, and I did quite a lot of work to help my mother before I'd leave for work.

"One of my classmates, Scottie, was on duty with me on the medical floor, and she told me the night supervisor had said she could watch a delivery if there was one that night. I said, 'All right, if I happen to be off, let me know and I'll get up.' She said, 'Miss Oke, I've got the medicine poured and everybody washed.' This was 3 a.m.! 'I've got everything done. Miss Mann said if I came up now, I might be in time.' When we went to breakfast, Scottie hadn't come back. By and by she came down white as a sheet! 'I'm never going to get married and never going to have a baby!' The last I heard Scottie had six! She was one of the younger ones of our group.

"We weren't supposed to go out to visit, and I never visited much to tell the truth. I would visit Anne Boyd who lived on Long Island, but I didn't make many outside friends. We weren't Baptists but four or five of us would go to the Baptist Temple Sunday after Sunday. They had a lovely service and afterwards they served doughnuts and coffee in a lovely parlour with an open fire. It was a home away from home. We loved it! And I had friends from Newfoundland not far from the hospital, but you didn't get much chance to loaf freely.

"After probation, we worked a twelve-hour day, seven days a week. We'd go on the wards two hours in the morning and in the afternoon, then we had classes for the rest of the day. I found night duty hard because I couldn't sleep in the day and I couldn't eat a dinner when I got up! I'd go visit my cousin, Flora, who didn't live far away and have tea and toast.

"Em Mifflin, my friend, had relatives not far from the hospital. We went there quite a lot. One day she said, 'We're going for a ride. What time have you got to be in?' I said, 'I applied for an eleven o'clock late leave.' We didn't get home until after eleven and they pulled the car right up to the Outpatients Department. Em and I walked through Outpatients and right into the night supervisor! We told her we were late because we'd been for a drive. We never heard a word about it, she didn't report us!

"We'd get old State Board papers, and a girl from Prince Edward Island, Anne Boyd, Em, and I would ask each other questions. That's how we studied for our State Boards. When the State Board results came in, Miss Heiner came up and said, 'Miss Oke, we've never experienced this before, but you have a 100% in Materia Medica. I had to come and tell you because they don't send the marks out.' I was very pleased and I will say she was really excellent!

"I didn't know much about the Depression because as students we got an allowance: ten dollars the first year, twelve dollars the next year, and fifteen the next year. When I graduated, we only got twenty-six cents on the dollar at home. I had to save for a uniform but I wouldn't send home for more money because I figured I'd probably get a present from my aunt and others. I got a nice bit of money and bought my uniform about six months before graduation but I didn't wear it. We wore our caps and a black band for the last six months. After I graduated, I got seventy a month for floor duty and had maintenance [room and board].

"After training, I had an interview with Miss Rogers, who was the Superintendent of Nurses. She said, 'Have you thought about the future?' and I said, 'Not too much but I would like to specialize in psychiatry.' She said, 'Miss Oke, I think that would be a very hard life for you. What is your next choice?' and I said, 'Children.' I stayed at the hospital and one morning, I was called to Miss Rogers' office. There was a nurse there from the Childs Hospital and she suggested I go to Albany to work and see if I could do better with my high school credits. I had gone back to school because I was only credited with a year and a half of high school, which was the requirement to go in training in the States. Spencer didn't give me credit for some courses because I didn't do CHE [public exams] in them. Spencer did put me down as having bacteriology, but if they had put down general science, I'd have been all right. The nursing school gave me credit for a business course and I also had matric, but I had to take American History. I also took English because I was fond of it. I'd write favour and savour and words with 'o-u-r.' The professor said, 'Look at Miss Oke's paper and tell me what's wrong there.' They all picked the wrong spelling. He said, 'Miss Oke comes from Newfoundland and that's the English teaching.' I tried school twice but gave it up both times because I did weeks and weeks of twelve-hour night duty, eleven weeks in one stretch. I was trying to go to school and work, and I had to give it up.

"Anyway I decided to go for an interview with Mr. Field at the Childs Hospital and wrote my friend, Peg Harvey in Albany, to get me a hotel room, but I got a phone call from the hospital to say I was to stay there with the Head Nurse. She and a friend met me and we went to dinner before going to the hospital. The next morning, this lovely white-haired person came, brought me a basin to wash and a tray. I was in one of the private rooms! After my interview with Mr. Field, I went back to St. John's Hospital and a few weeks later I received a letter saying they liked me at the interview and would I consider coming to Childs Hospital. I went to see Miss Rogers and she said, 'My dear, there's your chance and if you don't like it, you can always come back to us,' which was nice of her.

"That was 1934 and I went home for the summer. I joined the hospital in Albany in September. It was only an eighty-bed children's hospital but I loved it! The Childs Hospital was mainly for city children. It also had a summer hospital in Saratoga. We had a lot of polio patients there, and the first year I went to Saratoga, we had nineteen children on frames with polio or TB spines. We had a little Jewish boy, almost completely paralyzed, who played 'Silent Night' on the xylophone. We also had a patient who had surgery for spina bifida and did very well. You got very fond of these children because you were with them for a while.

"I was looking after an 18-month-old boy and said to the doctor, 'I think this little fellow needs attention right now.' The doctor asked, 'What do you think it is?' They'd ask me to see what I'd say because I'd stick out my neck. I said, 'I think he's got appendicitis.' He was in for surgery because he had an undescended testicle but he fussed so much that I said, 'I think there's more than that.' Anyway I scrubbed to assist at the operation and when the doctor cut the hernial sac, up popped a red-hot appendix. The doctor put down his tools because he really got a start! 'Have you ever considered how wonderful the dear Lord is?' he said. He probably saved the boy's life because he did the surgery then. I loved those children!

"The hospital also did a lot of drug experiments because the aspirin factory was just across the river from Albany in Windsor. We also had a few adult rooms which were used to test drugs. There was a girl trained to do urine and ordinary blood, but she couldn't do things like cross matching and I typed the x-ray reports. It was quite an interesting place and the doctors were wonderful.

"We were so busy making plasters, bandages, and gauze. We had a sterilizer and took care of all that, which was the same at the hospital where I trained. You never stopped a minute in the operating room; we did a lot of tonsillectomies. Patients were in bed for six and seven days and we had four rooms with a cot where the mother could stay with the child.

"We had excellent food there because Miss Clarke, the Head Nurse, and I ate with the Sisters! It was funny because we sat at their table and the students sat elsewhere and didn't get what we had. I didn't like that. The Sisters ate in the Sisters' House in the evening and we ate the same as the students.

"We had a wonderful board of managers who gave wonderful gifts to the children at Christmas. Just before the Christmas party, one little boy said, 'Miss Oke, you're my girlfriend, aren't you?' and I said, 'I hope so, Mikie, what's the matter?' He said, 'I've asked Santa Claus for a flashlight and I'd like to know if he will have one for me.' I said, 'Well, I'll talk to Santa Claus and see what I can do.' The party was the next day and the hospital put this beautiful big box on his bed, but Mikie just pushed it to the foot of the bed. Santa Claus came over and said, 'Mikie, how come you get a second package?' I had bought a flashlight and wrapped it up. Mikie peeled off the paper and said, 'Open your mouth until I look at your tonsils.' He wanted to play doctor!

"On one of our trips to the hospital in Saratoga, one of the children said, 'We're going to Saratoga and I haven't got a suitcase.' An Anglican Sisterhood was in charge of the hospital and I told this to Sister Lydia, the superintendent. She said, 'Get Miss Calhoun out of the operating room. I'll give you some money to get all the little suitcases you can.' We came back loaded down! The teachers got the biggest kick when one boy's suitcase fell open and he had nothing but a *National Geographic* magazine inside!

"I was Head Nurse at the Childs during the Second World War. We used to have air raid drills. And the doctor came over for the drill. One night Sister Lydia said to us, 'This would be different if it was the real thing.' Dr. Dodge told her, 'Don't say that, Sister, we're supposed to be practicing as if it were the real thing.' That's when I took my Red Cross course.

"We organized a training school for practical nurses and I designed their uniform. They affiliated with Glen Falls Hospital for baby training. I'm home since the early fifties and I still get cards on special occasions like Easter and Christmas from the alumni of that hospital. I've gone to a couple of banquets and after the last one in September 1986 a girl wrote me and said, 'Miss Oke, I came from California where I have been living since I got married. When I heard your name, it brought back memories of the second chance I was given in training.' She got into trouble and they wanted to drop her, but I thought she should be allowed to go home, have her baby, and then start again if she wished. She remembered that after all that time!

"I worked in Albany for ten years. Then I came back to Newfoundland and stayed for a year and a half. I did private duty for eight and a half months with Mrs. Percy Crosbie. I did a few cases at St. Clare's, the Grace, and the General, but I didn't like private duty. I liked to be really busy. I found the Childs Hospital the most interesting.

"I knew another Newfoundlander when I was in Albany, a Miss Blanche Pittman who was Principal of St. Agnes School. I got a letter from her while I was home, telling me that the school nurse was leaving to be married and she wondered if I would consider taking the nurse's place. I went there in January as the school nurse and I enjoyed that. I had a kitchen and a bed-sitting room. I had a car most of the time and could go around Albany on my time off because it was within four mountain ranges and very lovely. I had lots of social life then.

"St. Agnes was a country day school with 50 boarders from well-to-do families. There was an infirmary for students who got sick and I inspected the students every morning. It was a different type of child health care because we also took them into town for their teeth and dealt with things like menstrual disorders. Even though we had a housemother, I dealt with homesickness. Miss Pittman would say, 'There's a few homesick ones up there. Take them for a ride and I'll give you money to get them an ice cream.' I had to take my turn chaperoning the students in town, so I had a chauffeur's license because I couldn't drive the children without it. Friday afternoon was a half-day and we'd take the students into town and have a big scoff at Hailey's Restaurant, or on Sunday afternoons we'd take them for drives in the school bus."

After her mother's death, Miss Oke returned to St. John's to be with her sister and didn't return to nursing.

CHAPTER 6:

Charlotte Somerton

*"We got a day off whenever it was convenient for the floor.
Whoever was in charge made up the list, put it on the desk,
and we were expected to check it. If we didn't, the supervisor
said we weren't very interested. If we missed taking our time
off it was seen as our fault and we didn't get another day off.
If we had to go to the residence to get something, the time it took
to go and come back was taken off our free time."*

Charlotte Somerton [Pomeroy] was born in Portugal Cove in 1904
but grew up on Bell Island when the iron ore mines were in
production and the local economy thriving. Her stories tell of the
lifestyle enjoyed on Bell Island in that day. Charlotte graduated
from the Grace Hospital in 1932 and remained there as a surgical
nurse for the majority of her working career.

When she was five, Charlotte's family moved to Bell Island.
"We had a wonderful life. That is the only way I can describe it,
perfect! We had plenty to eat, drink, plenty of clothes, and money
when we wanted it. Dad had a good job and we were never
wanting for anything. The merchants got in their winter supplies in

October because once the ice came in it stayed until June. But people weren't stuck because they had plenty. Each fall, they'd buy a 42-pound or a 10-pound tub of butter according to their circumstances. Everybody lived a wonderful life.

"My father worked for the Dominion Iron and Steel. He didn't work in the mines, he serviced the cars when they came up from underground. He had between 75 and 100 men. He worked hard and had a big responsibility with practically no wages. He came home one day and told my mother, 'I got an increase today.' And she said, 'How much are you getting an hour?' He got fifty cents an hour for 18 hours a day in the summer when the boats came in with the ore: $9.00 a day. Only five or six men on the island got that much money. It was a big job. Dad worked there 50 years. My brother got his job when Dad retired and was working in the mines when they closed in 1952 or '53 but then men were only working two days a week.

"My mother worked hard. She knit, sewed, patched, and did everything a housewife would do. She went to the church association one night a week. She joined the Orange Association, which meant she was out two nights a week. My mother had a full-time job, and if I could do anything for her, I did it. My father was an Orangeman and he'd go out one night a week. He belonged to the lodge in Portugal Cove, but sometimes by the time he'd get home from work, get the iron ore washed off, and put on clean clothes, he wouldn't be able to go.

"I wanted to join the tennis club but you had to be *somebody* to get in. We couldn't play tennis during the day but if we joined we could go to the dances and parties. People said, 'Don't be so foolish, you're not going to get in.' I said to my friend, 'Let's put in an application and see if we can get in.' She said, 'It's a waste of time,' and I said, 'There's nobody up there any better than I am except maybe financially.' So we put in an application. One day the tennis club president came in the shop and said, 'I've got good news, you and Reese got in.' Well the crowd nearly fainted! They had a Valentine's party like they do now and we enjoyed it to the full! I skated a lot but you could curl and do whatever sport you wanted. They played hockey in the winter and taught football in summer. There was always something to do. It was a wonderful life on Bell Island.

"I graduated from school at 15 and worked in a shop about eight years. Four of us worked for the Cowen family who were wonderful people to work for! I enjoyed ever minute in the shop. I would rather work with a Jewish person for $5 a month than work with a Newfoundlander for a $105. Every Saturday evening we'd stay for tea, and Mrs. Cowen always had baked beans and brown bread with caraway seed. That was their regular meal.

"I had two brothers in the First World War; both came back. One was in the navy for a year and a half. He came home on leave and could have gotten an honourable discharge but he joined the Regiment and went back over. He was badly wounded in the July 1st offensive and came home after the war. My oldest brother wanted to go to war too but they wouldn't take him. My aunt had three sons killed in that war, terrible!

"I wanted to do nursing all my life. I often said to Mom, 'Nursing is like running around behind the counter.' It just came in my mind one day and another girl in my class was going. My mother and father were delighted for me to go.

"Everyone except one girl in our class failed anatomy and she studied all the time. Eight failed so they made up another paper and everybody passed. Oh, my God! The papers, the muscles! The professor came from Memorial one night a week for chemistry. Everyone found that hard too but anatomy was the worst. We went to Memorial one night a week for diet clinic with Miss Penny, the dietitian. We each had our little desk and whatever we made, we could take home.

"As a probie, we wore an apron, which had to be a certain length, but no bib. You had to have your own scissors which came from the mainland with your name engraved on it. You got them when you got your apron. You also had to have red and blue ballpoint pens; red was used on nights... After three months we wrote an exam and if we passed we got the bib. Then three months later we wrote another exam and got our cap. When we went to breakfast, the Director of Nurses would stand at the foot of the stairs and as we went up the stairs, if she saw our stockings rolled we lost our half-day of free time. The uniforms were comfortable but the collars chafed your neck. Some wore their collars for weeks and they'd be so brown from perspiration. Same with the cuffs, they weren't always the cleanest! We only wore sleeves when we worked on the floors but we had to wear cuffs when you went to meals. That was a part of the uniform. The cuffs were left in the utility room and whoever went to the first meal got first pick. One girl never had a pair of cuffs; she always wore cuffs belonging to somebody else.

"We did a lot of house cleaning in nursing. The entrance to the ward was washed and polished before the doctors made rounds at nine each morning. We washed walls at least every month but we didn't do the floors. Utensils were cleaned every day of the week but Sunday. We washed the caseroom laundry and the padholders (a piece of cloth used as a binder), which also had to be scalded to get them clean. I asked for a T binder one time when I worked with private patients at St. Clare's, and Sister said, 'You're from the Grace, aren't you? I thought so because we don't use them here.' To me, pinning the pads onto the binder made the patients more comfortable.

"As students, we did everything from giving an enema to a drink of water. We did everything for men and women because we had no orderlies. We bathed patients but only private patients were bathed every day. All other patients were bathed in turn. Patients who had surgery had a full bed bath every morning for five or six days after the operation, then every second morning. After appendix surgery, a patient was in bed nearly two weeks and washed every day until the stitches came out. I only saw one patient get a shampoo, an old lady who had a private duty nurse who recently finished training in Montreal. The nurse got a Kelly pad, put the patient's head in it and the rubber part over the bed into the pail. Then she brought in a big pitcher of water which ran down into the pail. She did a wonderful job; it was something to see. I'll never forget it! It came to her as easy as giving a drink of water.

"I was going to leave nursing once after a night when we had a lot of deliveries, one after the other. There wasn't a pair of rubber gloves for dear life and everything was so dirty it would turn your stomach! Miss Oakley was in charge of the caseroom with Miss Thomas, and she kept bringing out pails of caseroom clothes. We had to wash blood out of everything and it was the hardest kind of work! I thought to myself, 'This is the last one. I am not washing any more of these and when I finish I'm going home.' I went to see the nurse who was in charge of the nursery and she said, 'Where are you going?' I told her, 'I'm going home.' She said, 'What happened?' and I told her, 'I can't do another pail of caseroom clothes or I'm gone!' She said, 'You won't get another one today.' So I said, 'All right I'll wait until tomorrow and see what happens.' That was the only time I was really going home. It was hard work!

"We worked 12 hours from seven to seven, seven days a week with one half day off each week. We didn't have much time off in that twelve hours; only one hour a day if we had two classes and two hours a day if we had one class. We got a day off whenever it was convenient for the floor. Whoever was in charge made up the list which was ready by 10 a.m. It was put on the desk and we were expected to check it. If we didn't, the supervisor said, 'We weren't very interested.' If we missed taking our time off it was seen as our fault and we didn't get another day off. If we had to go to the residence to get something, the time it took us to go and come back was taken off our free time. If we wanted to go anywhere special we had to ask permission a day or two before. If you wanted Friday off instead of Thursday somebody would always change with you, but you didn't ask for that very often unless it was something really special.

"We had to be in by ten o'clock and we had one late leave until eleven o'clock each week. When we had one or two hours off during the day, we'd run downtown because the stores closed at five or six o'clock. There were no buses but we usually drove back in one of the taxis on Waldegrave Street. We got $7.00 a month. One girl paid for her books out of that and books were expensive! Some months they'd take one dollar from her, and other months they'd take seventy-five cents. Out of that $7.00, we paid ten cents each to get our caps, collars, and coats done. But every Monday Mom sent me $5.00 or $10.00 pocket money in a parcel and my parents clothed me. We had plenty to do socially, as much as you could keep up with. Some girls went dancing like on New Year's Eve. We skated on Mundy Pond but I was the only one with boots and skates, and the girls would say, 'You're on night duty. How about lending us your boots and skates?'

"There was a shop across from the hospital where we could buy a pound of boiled ham for thirty or forty cents and get tomatoes in the summer. There was never enough food but we weren't starved! Breakfast was 6 a.m. and you got porridge or sometimes toast but not often because it took too much butter to have toast every morning. Some mornings we got a slice of bologna and others we'd have brewis. Every Monday was corn beef and potatoes, sometimes with lima beans or something like that. Every Sunday evening for 52 weeks we got a slice of bully beef and applesauce. In the summer, we might have lettuce with it. One evening a week we'd get a baked potato, a half one if it was large or a whole one if it was small. One of the nurses lived across the field from the hospital, and she would bring a few tea buns or something when she came back to residence at night and we'd have it with a cup of tea. Her mother was a wonderful baker. There was a lot of comradeship. We'd sit in the faculty sitting room and sing and play. It was wonderful! Everybody was happy. Nursing is a wonderful profession, that's the only way I can describe it. I enjoyed every minute of it. There isn't five minutes when I say I was unhappy while I was in training. We had lots of fun.

"I had a good preparation when I started as a graduate nurse. I was proud of my training. I worked on a surgical ward after I graduated. If there was an accident, patients stayed at the Grace if they had a broken leg, but if it was serious or the patient severely broken up they were immediately transferred to the General Hospital because they had more equipment than the Grace or St. Clare's. We did a lot of mastoid operations, gallbladders, appendix, and kidney removal, much the same as now and they did good work, I must say. For a few days before surgery, gastrectomy patients had milk and cream only. Then, after surgery, they had milk so many days, cream soup so many days, then broth but nothing heavy. They stayed in bed until they got their stitches out, which might be 10 or 12 days later. Then you got them out and put them back in bed two or three times a day. It was hard work! It was hard on the patient and breaking up your body too. I think that's why so many staff got hernias. Of course if Patten saw you trying to get a patient out of bed alone you lost your half time or free time.

"I had hundreds of maternity patients because I did night duty for six months. We didn't do deliveries alone as a student, but if a patient came in two or three in the morning you didn't have much chance to get a doctor, although Dr. Carter would come in at 2 a.m., stand at the front entrance, take a couple of tins of sausages or sardines out of his pocket, and have a cup of tea. Then he was ready to go! If a mother came in you'd help her wait until the doctor came, but you always knew if it was an emergency. There was no prenatal care in those days. The women came to hospital when they were due, although most were booked to come in. They weren't out of bed for nine or ten days after they delivered, only to walk to the bathroom. They weren't allowed to do anything. We washed their face and hands for the first three days. Nobody mentioned going home until their time was up and everybody breast-fed; it was compulsory. They'd send a sample of milk to the lab to get it tested, and if it were all right they'd take the baby out to the mother to nurse. Many of the mothers were poor and didn't have very much. I brought home more nightdresses to wash because most only had one nightdress. I'd bring it home in the evening, wash it, and take it back clean in the morning. We'd put a Johnny coat on them for the night. Miss Thomas was a supervisor and she had a box in case a baby needed things to go home. She used to call it the poor box. Miss Thomas was outstanding. She came up one morning about 2 a.m. A woman had died and Miss Thomas was crying. She said, 'We have no clothes to put on her.' I had a silk, hand-worked nightdress that I got for Christmas. I said, 'Miss Thomas, I have a nightdress in the drawer and I've never had it on,' so I gave it to her. Somebody gave her a pair of pants and another girl gave her a pair of stockings. You wouldn't know but someone had given Miss Thomas a million dollars because she had something to put on the patient.

"We had plenty of patients with pneumonia. They were treated with mustard plaster and linseed meal folder. You would rub olive oil on the skin, put the linseed meal poultice between gauze, then put the mustard plaster on the patient and keep watch. If the skin got red you discontinued it because they could get burned with the mustard plaster. One night Dr. Jameson was making rounds and went to see a sick baby in a house on King's Bridge Road. He asked the mother if she knew how to make a mustard plaster and she said, 'Yes.' He said, 'Because if you don't I'll tell you how to do it,' but she said she knew how to make it. On his way home he suspected she didn't know but didn't want to tell him, so he went back to see how she got along. He said, 'Did you get the linseed mustard plaster made?' and she said, 'Yes.' He said, 'I'll have a look before I go.' When he took off the baby's pajamas she had covered his little body with prepared mustard! Dr. Jameson said, 'Why don't you double him up and make a sandwich out of him.' [laughing]

"We didn't have antibiotics in our day. If a patient had a fever you gave him tepid sponge baths two or three times a day and plenty of fluids. We had aspirin with codeine and it was up to the nurse in charge to decide if a patient needed it. She couldn't prescribe but if I said a patient had pain, she would say, 'Give them Empirin or Empirin with codeine if it continues.' If there was more than one patient in the room where you were taking the pill you might as well take one for everyone because they would have one in minutes. Sometime we'd give them a needle with sterile water, which was one way to know if they had pain or not or whether it was just in their mind. If the pain continued we gave them Empirin with codeine. K9 [analgesic] was stronger than Empirin but only the doctor prescribed that. Nine times out of ten the doctor would leave the order and tell the nurse in charge she could use her judgment. Drugs came from the dispensary but there weren't many drugs on the go then. We had K9s, morphine sulphate, and sodium carbonate tablets for patients with gas. There were always two nurses on medications and when you took the bottle out of the cupboard you checked it and checked it again before you put it back. There were seven or eight nurses on the floor in the daytime and two on at night, because there weren't many patients out of bed at nighttime, but there was no guarantee you'd find another nurse at night. One nurse did x-rays. We weren't taught how to do them but she was. We tested urine in the lab. Nursing covered everything then.

"As far as I am concerned, nursing was perfection. You could do whatever you wanted as long as you did it well. One of the girls was going to do public health around the bay and one morning during a lecture, Dr. Roberts said to her, 'You're going to an outport. You've been shown what to do, and what you've been taught, do well. If you go out there thinking you can do doctor's work or that you can do everything, you will be a complete failure, sure enough.' He was trying to tell her to do what she was taught in the hospital and that was all that was expected of her."

CHAPTER 7:

Bertha Roberts

"We were on night duty at 7 p.m. and if
we were lucky we got off at seven in the morning.
You didn't get off until everything was done."

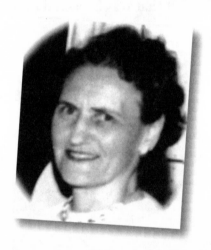

Bertha Roberts was born in Valleyfield, Bonavista Bay, in 1910 but moved to St. John's as a young girl. She graduated from the General Hospital in 1933 and was awarded the Harry J. Crowe Award for first place in class. Following graduation, Miss Roberts completed a dietetics course at the Halifax Ladies College, followed by an obstetrics course at the Halifax Infirmary.

Miss Roberts practiced primarily as a staff nurse in a variety of clinical settings throughout her career.

Bertha Roberts entered nursing in August 1929. "I liked caring for people and have never regretted it. As a matter of fact I wouldn't mind doing my training over. There were nine in my class and we joined the class who started six months before us. Miss Taylor taught general nursing and we had lectures from doctors in anatomy, medicine, pediatrics and drugs and surgery. Doctor Keegan gave ten lectures in surgery and we had to remember what he told us! By the end I could read his lectures off verbatim because he was interesting and you remembered it.

"In training we worked seven days a week. We went on night duty at 7 p.m. and if we were lucky got off at seven in the morning. You didn't get off until everything was done. We ate dinner at six o'clock before we went on duty. From eight to nine o'clock was visiting hours and at nine all the patients had their backs washed. We removed patients' many-tailed binders, rubbed their backs, and settled everyone for the night. At four in the morning, we repeated this ritual of taking off binders, rubbing backs, washing faces, cleaning teeth, and getting everyone ready for breakfast. These were the routines that happened at night. When we went off duty, we had breakfast. I was on Carson, which was a septic ward with only one nurse on from 10 a.m. to 2 p.m. and she had to do about 14 to 15 dressings each morning. By the time you got all the dressings done, you didn't have much time. Then you had to set up trays for dinner, serve dinner, tidy beds, and sweep the ward before the night staff came on. We had a lot of duties besides nursing but the patients got looked after. It wasn't nursing; it was manual labour!

"I was on duty one night when an old man got out of bed and tried to cut my throat. I was relieving the nurse on the ward who was outside doing something. I was making sponges and dressings and I knew nothing until the man had me by the shoulders. He had a long open razor and was going to finish me. I was between two beds and couldn't do much. I called the nurse but she didn't hear me. Everybody on the ward was asleep except a man who had an appendix operation that day. He tried to get out of bed but fell on the floor and I couldn't do anything for him. Miss Taylor heard me calling and then an orderly came. They put a strait-jacket on the man. I suppose he was confused. I wasn't frightened because I'm ready to go anytime one way or the other!

"The day staff came on at seven and made beds until they served breakfast at eight o'clock. We had no time off in the morning. At ten o'clock each morning the sick patients had chicken or beef broth or eggnog according to their illness. When a patient came in who was undernourished, Dr. Copperthwaite would say, 'What ward is Roberts on?' Because every time he saw me I had something on a tray to feed a patient, so he would tell them to send the undernourished ones to me. The poor fellows never had much and the poorer they were, the more attention I gave them.

"I went to the Fever Hospital in my first year as a possible typhoid fever, and they put me in a room with two typhoid patients, which was nice. I wasn't there very long. At night they brought around a cold stew or something cold in a bowl, but I never had it because you weren't supposed to eat too much with typhoid fever. Two people gave you a bath, one on each side of the bed. One washed down, the other washed the opposite way and that was your bath! They told me I had the funniest chart they ever saw because my temperature would go up to a hundred and three sometimes and I had a lot of pain with typhoid, although they didn't believe me. They'd say, 'You're not suppose to have pain with typhoid fever,' and so they didn't think I had any pain. I don't think they ever gave me anything for pain but I survived! I went home for two weeks after the typhoid fever, which was counted as my first-year holidays. I had no more holidays until my second year when I got another two weeks. Then in my third year I went home because my sister was there. We always had somebody sick in the family and I was the one who cared for them. Mom took advantage of me.

"I was in nursing when they had that tidal wave on the south coast in 1929. At first we thought it was thunder or something on the roof and the dishes started to rattle, but that was all we felt of it. There were homes and lives lost but it didn't affect us.

"Residence wasn't too bad. First when we moved in we shared a room but then we had a room to ourselves. The old residence was not very clean, so I cleaned every room I had. They used to say, 'If we move you around enough we'll get the whole place cleaned!' We moved to another room when we came off night duty and the one I got was filthy. Mary Carney said, 'I'll help you wash the walls.' We were having a grand time when in walked Miss Taylor! She sent Mary to her room and said everything to me about cleaning the room. I said, 'Miss Taylor, I'm not going to bed until this is cleaned!' It wasn't a nurse's job, but I always cleaned the rooms I had and the maids would come to clean the floors.

"Miss Taylor was very strict. We had to be in residence by half past ten if we went out, but we got a late leave once every two weeks until twelve o'clock. Sometimes it might be until one o'clock. I'd say, 'Miss Taylor, I'd like to stay out tonight.' And she'd say, 'Do you want late leave?' I'd say, 'No!' because I wanted to keep my late leave for my day off. I'd say, 'I only want to stay out until midnight.' She'd look at me with her black eyes but she'd let me go. I really got along well with her.

"We had very little time off so we didn't do much except go to an occasional show. There was no bus service so we made our own fun. Those interested in boys had boyfriends. We were off from 7 p.m. to 10 p.m. each day and had one day off every two weeks. But you didn't always get off at 7 p.m. Sometimes you'd be called back to the operating room if anything happened at night. If you were called back, you could be there until four in the morning but still had to be on duty at seven. A little thing like working late didn't make any difference. On Sundays, the Protestant girls worked every morning and the Catholic girls were off 10 a.m. to 2 p.m. to go to church. We worked from 7 a.m. until 2 p.m. when they came back on and we could go to church when we got off, if we wanted to.

"The food for the nurses was terrible. We had square biscuits for lunches at night which we called stomach shingles. Sunday morning we'd have beans, and other mornings we'd have cereal or toast and bacon. Dinner at noon was always a cooked meal but we seldom had anything other than cold suppers. I came over to the residence around 4 p.m. one day and one of the girls said, 'Roberts, we have a lovely supper tonight!' I said, 'What have we got?' 'Steak,' she said. Out came a nice piece of steak on a plate with nice brown gravy. I took my steak, turned it over, and underneath was a great big fly. She said, 'Aren't you going to eat it?' I said, 'I couldn't!' So she took it and ate it! I couldn't eat it even if I hadn't eaten anything for years! For a cold supper we'd have macaroni and cheese or shepherd's pie. I ate so little! Sometimes I went home to eat because the residence wasn't very clean and I was used to cleanliness. When we were on night duty we'd get a stew or something like that. I went to the kitchen a lot because I was always looking for something to eat but the kitchen wasn't very clean. There were no screens and we had this old tanglefoot hanging everywhere in the kitchen and the flies would stick to it. I offended a doctor who was giving us a lecture about sterilization because I said, 'Sterilization and nobody bothers to put screens up for the flies!'

"If there was anything that shouldn't be there, I was the one that found it. First when I went in training I was on duty one day and serving the soup. I stirred it and there were spiders in it, so I took the soup and threw it down the sink and a lot of patients didn't get soup for their dinner! They heard in the kitchen that I threw out the soup and someone said, 'Miss Roberts, you won't last here.' I said, 'If I wouldn't drink it myself, I wouldn't give it to the patients.' Anyhow I didn't hear any more about it and I didn't see any more spiders!

"We had gallbladders, cancer of the bowel, appendix, broken bones – the usual things. We had a lot of pneumonia, which was a lot of work because we put a linseed poultice on the patient. We made it up and had it very hot. Then we put the poultice between two pieces of material with a bandage over it to keep it warm. Then put it on the patient's chest and changed it every four hours. I don't know whether it helped them or not, I can't say. Pneumonia patients also got lots of fluids. They would be listless but most of them got better except older patients. We didn't have antibiotics then but we did before I left nursing. At that time, we had M&B 693 pills and morphine, and we gave heroin by injection if patients had a lot of pain. We'd sterilize the needle with the old burner. Nurses did everything then.

"Getting patients ready for an operation was quite a ritual. How many times would you have to wash the patient before surgery! You'd sterilize the bowls, sponges, and anything else you'd need. You wore rubber gloves and washed the patient with green soap, then put sterile towels around them. The next morning all that came off and you repeated the same ritual. Then you painted the patient with gentian violet, iodine or mercurochrome – whatever they were using. Someone told an orderly to paint a patient with iodine and when they checked, the patient was painted from his neck to his thighs. They didn't know but he was a Red Indian. [laughing]

"I was afraid of nobody, not even Dr. Keegan, although most people were. He was a tall man, and it would put the fear of God in you to look at him. He was very particular and if the interns weren't on duty by quarter to eight, they'd get it. If he told you to do something he expected it to be done and if it wasn't...[laughing]. He'd come in at night to see stomach cases. We gave them soup and Bengal's Food at night and they'd come to me from other wards to make the Bengal Food and soup. Bengal's Food was a powder we mixed with milk. Dr. Keegan would say, 'Never tell a patient they can't have anything.' But that was difficult because the kitchen was locked at night, and if somebody woke up in the middle of the night and wanted something, well what were you going to do because everything was locked up!

"I graduated in 1933, but we didn't have a graduation ceremony. We just finished! Nobody ever said, 'Congratulations!' You went to the office and were given your graduation pin. We also got a diploma but I lost mine. But nobody thought much about graduation then. I got the Harry J.Crowe scholarship for coming first in my class, but I don't know if that was much of an achievement or not. There were those who said I hadn't worked for it, and I knew I hadn't worked for it. One girl in the class wanted it, and as a matter of fact, I would have given it to her. There was quite a bit of jealousy in our class but we were friends!

"The nine of us who started nursing together did not finish on the same day because some had sick days added on and couldn't finish. I only lost two shifts when I was on nights, and apart from that I didn't have any sick time. None of us stayed on at the hospital, we went our different ways. In the fall of 1933, I started a course in dietetics at the Halifax Ladies College. I did two years in the one, which was a lot of hard work, but I enjoyed the course. It was quite an experience. I also went to the Halifax Infirmary for obstetrics because it wasn't part of my training. I could have gone to the Grace but I went to Halifax for a change. The nun told me I could come back if I wanted to. She said, 'Don't bother to send a message, just come on!' She told me I'd make a good nun but I said, 'Oh no! I'm not religious enough.' She said, 'That doesn't matter.

That will come.' I really enjoyed it there.

"I left the General in 1942 to do private duty nursing. Miss Rogers had worked at the General Hospital for a while and she asked me to come to Trois Rivieres in Quebec. I went for a change and worked at the French hospital there. It was quite interesting. The patients were French-speaking but most could also speak English. Unfortunately I didn't speak French. The French patients would say the English nurses were better than the French nurses because the French nurses made the patients get up and wash themselves the day after surgery. The French nurses didn't give them much care, but we got along with the French girls and they all spoke English. I was there a year when my mother got real sick and I came back to St. John's.

"I mostly did private duty nursing at St. Clare's. Sister would call me if they had a crooked patient and say, 'Miss Roberts, I've got a lovely patient for you.' This patient had been at the General and had nine nurses while he was there. He was too crooked for anybody to look after! So I said, 'Oh yes, Mr. Greene is a lovely patient!' Sister said, 'You can get along with people, can't you?' And I said, 'I'll try.' I think he had prostate cancer and he was crooked but I had no trouble with him. He'd have nightmares and wake up and refuse to sleep.

"I worked with another private duty nurse who was never on time. I did day duty and she was never there at four o'clock and the patient said to me one day, 'The other nurse always gets off on time, but you always have to wait for her. What's wrong with you that you can't get off?' Surprisingly, he kept her on. Sometimes I came on half past seven and the first thing he'd want was a cup of tea before his breakfast, but that wasn't easy to get because the hospital didn't have facilities as they have now.

"Most of my patients were cooperative but I had one patient, and when I came on my shift, the nurse who had been on with her said, 'Thank goodness you've come! I can't do anything with her. She was operated on yesterday and won't let anybody do anything.' I said, 'Give me the bed linen.' I went in and said, 'You don't look very comfortable.' 'I'm not,' she said. Evidently, she had gone to the operating room for a D&C but they did a hysterectomy and she was very annoyed! Rightly so! I said, 'I'll give you a bath and clean your bed and I think you'll feel better.' There were three nurses on with her and after about five days she said, 'I'm going to let one of my nurses go because she doesn't seem happy, but you don't seem to mind me.' I said, 'No! If a patient is uncooperative, I always think it's their illness, not their general personality. So it doesn't bother me.' She didn't say much to that.

I was on evenings with her and when I came on, the day nurse said, 'She's got to have her catheter changed.' I said, 'Why didn't you do it?' She said, 'I couldn't do that.' The patient had a vaginal hysterectomy and being catheterized wasn't very comfortable, so I called the doctor to see if I could give her something. I told her I was going to remove the catheter but would give her a needle first in case it bothered her. She said, 'I'm not having anything to do with that.' I said, 'All right, that's your prerogative.' I explained to her about Foley catheters and that I would have to take out the water in it before I removed it. I turned to get the syringe and she took the catheter and pulled it out. Why she didn't injure herself, I'll never know! She said, 'I thought you were going to give me a needle?' 'Well,' I said, 'it's not much good to give it to you now!' Anyway, I put in the new catheter and she said, 'That didn't hurt at all.' I tell you, she was crooked! But maybe she was justified, seeing as they did the surgery without her consent.

"I'm not into anything or go to anything in nursing now because I am really disillusioned with the profession. There are only two things on their minds, time off and pay. Nothing else matters."

CHAPTER 8:

Jennie Wareham

*"I always had a spirit of adventure and I wasn't going
to stay in Newfoundland if there were other fields to conquer.
I thought if I went to Montreal I could get my RN
and would have greater opportunities in nursing and broader
experiences than if I stayed at home."*

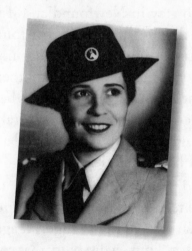

Jennie Wareham [Lauentius Burton] was born in Spencer's Cove,
Placentia Bay, in 1912. A self-proclaimed adventurer, Jennie
traveled to St. John's for high school and university before
entering nursing at the Montreal General Hospital. While doing

a postgraduate course in tuberculosis nursing after graduation, Jennie decided to participate in a nursing exchange with the South African government, a decision that would more than satisfy her spirit of adventure.

At the age of eight, Jennie Wareham moved with her family to Harbour Buffett. She left there to complete her schooling at Bishop Spencer College and Memorial College in St. John's before entering nursing at the Montreal General Hospital in 1931. "My mother influenced my decision to go in nursing because she was gifted as far as nursing was concerned. She was the person in the community who always knew what to do and I was always interested in what she was doing. I think she wanted me to be a nurse. My godmother had gone to the Montreal General and I felt if she could go there so could I! Besides, you couldn't get an RN (license) in St. John's, and I always had a spirit of adventure and I wasn't going to stay in Newfoundland if there were other fields to conquer. I thought if I went to Montreal I could get my RN and have greater opportunities in nursing and broader experiences than if I stayed at home. My mother was very happy but my father thought I should go to St. John's because the clergy-man's daughter trained at the St. John's General, and he thought what was good enough for the clergyman's daughter, was good enough for me. But I had other ideas."

Jennie possessed two of the admission requirements for nursing, grade 11 and references from her clergyman, but it was the medical certificate that created a challenge. At age two, Jennie had polio and was left with a "limp," a disability that could have kept her out of nursing. Not to be deterred, Jennie took measures to lessen that likelihood. "I persuaded the doctor who examined me in St. John's not to mention my disability and let me fight my problem when I got there, because I was afraid they would turn me down if they knew beforehand. I got in but two days after I was there, I was walking down a long corridor and the instructor behind me noticed I was a bit lame. She said, 'Miss Wareham, there's something wrong with your foot!' I said, 'Miss McKenzie, there's nothing wrong with my foot. I have a sore toe.' 'Don't you lie to me,' she said. 'You come with me to Miss Holt.' She was the Director of Nursing, and I immediately thought I'd have to go home but Miss Holt was very fair. She wasn't cross with me but she did say, 'You shouldn't do something like that!' I said, 'Miss Holt, I've wanted to be a nurse since I was six and wanted to come to the Montreal General. You can't send me home without giving me a chance!' So she said, 'All right, but go to the orthopedic specialist, and if he thinks you can be a nurse, we will give you the opportunity.' The doctor decided I could stay but I had to have physiotherapy throughout my training and I did. Many times I wished I hadn't chosen nursing because I was very tired but I managed well. The physiotherapy helped a lot. I went once a week and more often when my foot was really bothering me. It wasn't easy having a disability but it wasn't difficult either. I don't think I was any more tired than the others; we were all tired.

"It didn't cost much to get ready for nursing. I had to pay for my passage and uniforms which I took with me. Our textbooks were supplied but we had to give them back. They housed and fed us but we didn't get paid for three years! The idea was that we were becoming professionals and like other professionals, you paid for your education. The only money I had was what my mother sent, five dollars here and there, but we didn't need much because we didn't have time to spend it.

"I don't remember my first day in training because I was petrified I was going to be sent home and maybe I had a guilty conscience about being there. We were in a week when they took us to the floors from 7 to 9 a.m. and from 4 to 7 p.m. under the supervision of an instructor. Then we were in the classroom for the rest of the day. That lasted for the six months. We were called probies on probation and never allowed to forget it! Every day we were told, 'Don't think you're going to get through!' and we were scared to death because we thought we wouldn't make it and yet we were trying so hard. It was a terrible time because we were far from home and lonely but determined to get through! I will never forget those six months! We started with fifty-five and finished with thirty-three. Most left because they didn't make it in the exams or on the floors, and others left because they didn't like it or weren't interested. We were weeded out and told as much. Having a disability didn't make it any easier because it was always in the background. I always felt I had to make it and I did! Even though I was petrified, I loved every day of it!

"The worst part of that period was adjusting to being a probationer. We were less than dust to everybody from the second-year students up. We didn't dare get into the elevator with a second- or third-year student or a graduate. We could get on but not until they all got in first! We were allowed on the elevator only because we had to go up seven floors for meals. We weren't expected to walk seven floors, only one or two, and we did because we didn't have time to wait. I distinctly remember waiting twenty minutes outside the elevator to go for meals and then having only ten minutes left to eat. The third years considered themselves superior to the second-year students and probationers, and we were expected to look up to them and the graduates. But they were helpful and there was a good relationship between all of us. They demanded respect but we mostly felt awe!

"For most of our probation we were in the classroom. When we went to the floors in the morning, we helped with things like beds and breakfast. After classes, we went back from 4 to 7 p.m. and sometimes we didn't get off until 8 or later because all the work had to be finished before the night nurse came on, and we weren't allowed off until our work was done. If you had to spend another hour getting it done, too bad! Then we had homework for the next day but we tried to get to bed at ten or half past. I couldn't wake up at 6 a.m. and Miss McKenzie would say, 'Miss Wareham is three sheets to the wind!' because I was always nodding off and trying to keep my head up! I think she was taking it out on me because I lied to her about my limp.

"We had classes throughout training in subjects like biology, chemistry, bacteriology, anatomy and physiology, and nursing arts. The instructors, who were all McGill people with degrees and very qualified, taught these subjects. We were frightened to death of them but they were nice to us and we respected them. Margaret Batstone was a Newfoundlander and a perfectionist. She taught nursing arts and one day I was doing a milk and molasses enema when the tube came out. What a mess on the floor! I thought she was going to send me home. Many of our lectures in third year were given by doctors, but the instructors set the exams, which included demonstrations as well as oral and written exams.

"During probation, we wore a terrible uniform which was baggy and blue with a starched collar and cuffs and a long, white starched apron with black stockings and shoes. It never fit! Only graduates wore white shoes and stockings. When we passed the probation period and were accepted into nursing we had a capping ceremony. We still wore the blue uniform but it was fitted with a bib and we had our cap! It was a very insignificant looking cap! In third year, we wore a pink uniform with a pattern of the MGH letters on it. We were really proud of that!

"After those six months we were on the wards all day with three hours off for classes, usually 9 to 12 noon or 1 to 4 p.m. We had an instructor with us and weren't allowed to do anything we hadn't learned in the classroom and weren't proficient at. We did enemas and made beds, but bed making then was very specific, as was the bath! Patients were washed every morning, what the English called 'top and tail' but only had a bath once a week.

You covered them with a flannelette sheet, turned the bed linen down; and it took about an hour because we did their nails, toenails, ears, everything. The procedure was very specific and it took a long time to perfect it and do it properly. As students, we had no responsibilities, and when the girls came from South Africa on an exchange, they were horrified at how little we were permitted to do on our own. We couldn't give an aspirin without an order because MGH was a teaching hospital and the medical students needed the experience.

"We worked from 7 a.m. to 7 p.m. with three hours off when we usually had lectures. On Sundays we had five hours off and either worked from 7 a.m. to 2 p.m. or got off at two o'clock. We got one day off when we were in the diet kitchen or the operating room, but in the OR, you were always on call the night before your day off so it really didn't mean much. We spent our time off sleeping and that's how it was for three years! We didn't have sick leave as such, and if you did, you had to make it up but I didn't have any. I had treatment for my foot and it behaved well during training except I was always tired, but hard work never hurt anyone.

"Our social life didn't amount to much. We weren't allowed out during the week because we had to study. We could go out on weekends until 9:30 on a Saturday and 12 midnight once a month. Occasionally we'd go to a show but that wasn't often because we were too tired to go out anywhere. We weren't supposed to have boyfriends, but some girls did and they went out a bit more, and we weren't allowed to fraternize with the interns or medical students. I was very active in the Anglican Cathedral, which wasn't far from the hospital, and I belonged to the Student Christian Movement, which was affiliated with McGill. I met people there and I had an aunt in Montreal who I visited. There were seven Newfoundlanders in my class. Marion Sampson was a very close friend of mine, and Frieda Squires was at Memorial with me so we became friends.

Grace Mercer and I were friends at Memorial and Spencer, and I made friends with some others so it wasn't that lonely.

"We got two weeks holidays in the first and second year and I came home to Newfoundland. Most of the Newfoundlanders came home the same time. We came by boat, down the St. Lawrence to Charlottetown, St. Pierre, and St. John's. It took half my holidays to get home, but it was fun and my parents were delighted. One year, I had been on the private ward and gotten about ten boxes of chocolates and I brought them home. My family had a gorgeous time because chocolates were quite a treat in the '30s, but they could only have one at a time.

"The nurses' home was beautiful, seven stories with a lounge downstairs and a kitchen on each floor. Each class was housed on a certain floors; I was on the seventh. We had to be up and dressed, have our room tidy, be down to the elevator, through the tunnel and in the dining room on the seventh floor of the hospital by 20 minutes to seven each morning. If we weren't there, the door was locked and you didn't get any breakfast. An instructor was there to see that we had our hairnet and cap on properly. I could sleep through anything because I was always so tired. In my last two years, I was in the end room of the corridor and the fire alarm was outside my door, and I slept through the fire alarm! So I got one of those West alarm clocks, and I tied spoons, knives and things on it and put it over my head. It went off at quarter past six because six o'clock was too early for me, and I got up, got dressed and had my bed made in time, but if the housemother had opened my closet door during a room inspection, everything would have come down on top of her!

"Matron was an outstanding person and she was also in charge of the school. She had deep blue eyes that looked right through you and we were frightened to death of her, but she was fair. We had so much respect for her! She made rounds on the floors practically every day and knew exactly what was going on. She didn't speak to us unless she had something to say.

"We were scared to death of the doctors and wouldn't dare speak to them. Most treated us as if we didn't exist, especially the ones from McGill. They weren't unkind or anything, but we just didn't exist! McGill was a teaching hospital and the doctors had to teach the medical students so they didn't teach us on the floors. They paid a bit more attention to us in our third year because we were doing treatments. I guess the relationship was good because I don't recall any difficulty with them.

"Our affiliations were similar to those in other training schools. We had no responsibility in the affiliating hospitals; we were only there to learn. We had a couple of months in psychiatry and had marvelous psychiatrists like Dr. Vanier, who taught psychiatry at McGill and did amazing things. He hypnotized a girl, who had amnesia from a motor accident, for a half hour every day and went through her life, asking her questions. Eventually she got her memory back, which was really fascinating! We did three months maternity at the Royal Victoria and two months of infectious diseases at the Fever Hospital. The Montreal General had a pediatrics ward so we didn't go outside to affiliate and we did so many months in orthopedics, surgery, medicine, ten weeks night duty each year, six weeks in the diet kitchen, and time in the operating room at our own hospital.

"I learned French at Memorial, which didn't help me, but French wasn't a problem because we spoke English. Most people spoke English even in the Montreal shops so I gave up on it. We became friendly with the patients on the private wards and they understood English. We couldn't understand the maids and orderlies who were French because they spoke so rapidly. Many outpatients were French and we couldn't understand them either but we didn't have much contact with them. We had social workers who kept contact with the patients by going to their homes and making sure everything was okay.

"The Montreal General was located on Dorchester at St. Lawrence and Main, which was the worst part of Montreal. We were down in the slums and had the most amazing patient experiences. We had drug addicts because there were pushers on the street and I remember one young girl with a heroin addiction. We rehabilitated her but she came back a second time. It was very sad. I don't know what ever happened to her.

"We had a chap about twenty-four who was from Scotland and he had TB or what we called galloping consumption. It was terribly sad because he had no family and knew no one in Montreal. I stayed on duty until about nine o'clock to make him comfortable and do what I could for him because I knew he was going to die and felt somebody had to be close to him. He died that night.

"I remember the way we treated pneumonia. We had no medications so we used linseed meal poultices, sponges, and fluids and kept them warm. I remember going off duty, worrying about a patient who was terribly sick with a temperature of 104, then coming on duty the next morning to see the patient sitting up in bed with his temperature down to normal. It was something for a nurse to know it was only nursing care that kept them alive. It was very satisfying, no doubt about it! For me, it was one of the great satisfactions of nursing!

"I graduated in September 1934, but we didn't have much of a graduation ceremony. My mother and father took a week to come up by boat for the ceremony. We had afternoon tea in the lounge, and Matron and the administrator presented us with our diplomas and pins. We were very happy and very excited to think we got through three years. We felt it was quite an accomplishment! My father's sister was in Montreal so we went to Aunt Elsie's and had a big 'do' just for the family.

"I didn't stay at the MGH long after I graduated. I went to Western Hospital as a staff graduate and then on to Ste. Agathe in

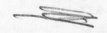

the Laurentians to do a six-month post-graduate course in TB nursing. The only treatment for TB then was fresh air, and there was plenty in the Laurentian Mountains. The patients spent most of their time outdoors with plenty of clothes, woolen caps on their head, and mitts, or indoors with the windows open. The patients were brought inside for care because it was too cold to expose them outside. They slept outdoors and most of the time they slept through the night. They used hot water bottles to keep warm, but mostly the patients were bundled up with lots of clothes. The bathrooms and bedrooms were heated but the windows kept open. The patients had good nourishment with plenty of milk, butter, and fats, but they didn't always have much appetite. There were no drugs and diet was the only treatment except for those who needed surgery. Patients were sent to Montreal for thoracoplasty surgery and came back when they were healed sufficiently. Pneumothorax treatments were done once a week or so. Patients who had pneumothorax or thoracoplasty done were miserable but the survival rate was surprisingly good. Only one older man died. The patients came from all parts of Quebec and their families weren't nearby so they seldom had visitors.

"While I was in the Laurentians I heard the South African government offered to exchange nurses with Canada for one year. Three of us applied to go and two were accepted. Clare Hiscock from Brigus went with me, but Helen Miller was not medically fit to go and I was! I wrote home that I wanted to go to South Africa and my family was astounded! Nobody knew much about South Africa and my father wanted to know more so he went to St. John's to see a friend who had been in the First World War. When he told Mr. Chafe I wanted to go to South Africa, he said, 'You can't let her do that! It's only jungle, a terrible place!' Pop thought it couldn't be that bad, so he had sense enough to go see Miss Cherrington, Principal of Spencer. When he told her I wanted to go to South Africa, she said, 'It's a beautiful country! I have a brother living in

Durban and he loves it. You must let her go.' That's how I got my parents' consent. They didn't mind me going because I had been in Montreal and was only going for a year. We had to get Canadian passports because the exchange was between Canada and South Africa, and as Newfoundland didn't have any immigration laws, we had to become Canadian citizens. We paid $200 for our fare and went on a cargo ship from Saint John, New Brunswick. The Montreal General gave us a farewell party and $200 each as a scholarship for pioneering! It was very thoughtful of them. Clare and I spent it on clothes because our families had already given us the money for our fare. We were paid $47.50 by the MGH that year, and the South African nurses were paid by their hospital in South Africa.

"Clare and I arrived in Cape Town on May 1, 1936. Clare went to work at Good Secour Hospital and I went to a cottage hospital in a suburb called Wynberg. The cottage hospital was very primitive with no medical students and only one doctor who came around once in a while. We didn't worry about what the doctor would do because we did everything. If a patient had a headache we gave the medications. I was there for a year – spent six months on a black ward and six months on a white ward. The white ward was in the same building, but the patients had it better than the blacks. The government was poor and the blacks suffered most. Patients on the black ward had sheets and pillowcases but no dressings. We'd tear up sterilized sheets and use them as dressings, but there was never any cross infection and the patients were happy with the treatment they got. We gave them the same nursing care we did the white people. The only difference was we didn't have the equipment we needed.

"Nurses' training in South Africa was also very primitive. On my first morning as a staff nurse on the black ward, the Sister in charge decided to teach me how to do dressings. She laid a sterile towel on the trolley, then took a large container from the shelf with scissors and things in it and the bottles she was going to use, and put them on the sterile towel! She said, 'I'll show you how to do a dressing.' She washed her hands when she started and that was the last time she washed them until she finished. She picked up the sterile things with her hands and I thought, 'What in the name of the Lord am I going to do?' because being in a strange country, you can't say, 'That's not the way to do it.' They'd resent it and they resented outsiders anyway. I was very careful and managed to keep things sterile without upsetting her. She didn't seem to resent it. On the white ward, things were better because the staff was more accomplished. I wanted to learn Afrikaans, but my Newfoundland and Canadian accents combined sounded peculiar, so when I spoke they'd laugh at my Afrikaans accent. I got shy about that and didn't learn it but I really didn't need it anyway.

"At the end of the year, we had no money to come back but we loved it and didn't want to come back. We got permission to stay but we had to sever our connections with the Montreal General. We had to decide what we wanted to do, so Clare stayed on as Nurse-in-Charge in the hospital but I wanted to do a Mother-Craft Training course in Cape Town. I did private duty with Jewish maternity patients and their babies. I would stay in their homes as part of the family for ten to fourteen days after delivery. I got fed on a case but had no money to eat in-between because I was saving for this maternity training. It was fun and I enjoyed it, and after three months I had enough saved to do the course. The theory behind the Mother-Craft Program was that every baby could be breastfed, regardless of any difficulties. Middle-class white people came to the home with babies who were difficult feeders and we got them back on an even keel. We did breast massage with hot and cold water, watched the mother's diet, and gave them lots of oatmeal water to drink and did certain exercises. We also gave the mother a supplement at the beginning and weighed the babies after every feed. We decreased the supplement as milk production increased and by three weeks most were fully breastfed. It was very interesting! I was on staff at the home for six months, and while I was there, they gave us time off to do public health lectures in the evenings. So I took public health, which in South Africa came under the Royal Sanitary Institute of England. Because I hadn't seen my parents since graduation, I decided I should go home but as usual I had no money, which was a chronic state of affairs! I went to Johannesburg in January 1939 because there was plenty of work, lots of rich people and better pay for private duty. I went with the idea of saving enough money to go home by March 1940, but in September 1939 war broke out, which is another story! I returned to Cape Town and volunteered for war service but the war was a long time starting in South Africa, so in the meantime, I joined the Health Department and did public health work in Cape Town among the natives and blacks.

"Public health in Cape Town was quite an experience. The people lived in hovels and homes under very primitive conditions with bugs, lice, and fleas. The blacks had come to the cities and put up whatever shelter they could. Their tribal homes were primitive so they were quite happy when they came to the city. The South African government put up housing developments but the people wouldn't go in them. At the end of each day, I'd go home, get undressed, stand in the bath, and let the fleas fall in the water. The most I counted was thirty-six! They were sand fleas and didn't bother you much except they were everywhere. My district was outside Cape Town and not very safe. I went by horse and cart and had a coloured man to guard me because of the bad elements, but the people respected a white person with a nurse's uniform, so I felt safe as long as I had this old coloured man with me. I did child welfare, and breastfeeding was part of public health because it was the safest way to feed the babies. We'd visit ten days after the baby was born and try to get the mothers and babies to come to the clinic. There was a lot of VD, and the aim was to look after the babies and treat the mothers for VD. While they were pregnant, we could force them by law to receive treatment, which meant the baby would be born disease free, but once the baby was born we couldn't do that. We wanted the mothers to continue treatment for VD but they could please themselves if they came or not. I had a bad incident where a man nearly pushed me down the stairs because I wanted his wife to come to the clinic after the baby was born. He said it was none of my business if his wife had VD so I had no choice but to leave her. Most of the black women weren't married and had children one after the other with very little control. They were immune to things that we weren't immune to because of their living conditions, but they were fairly healthy. It was survival of the fittest! The babies were beautiful with big black eyes and I loved doing baby clinics.

"I did public health for two years until I was called up in April 1941 and was sent to a military hospital in Johannesburg until November 1941. I went to the recruiting office and the doctor noticed one leg was shorter than the other and decided not to pass me. I said, 'Look, I've been walking the hills of Cape Town doing public health, which were much like the hills of St. John's. I can do whatever has to be done in the army.' I felt I could do ordinary duty and it wasn't going to be any worse than what I had been doing. But she still wouldn't pass me. I knew the recruiting officer in Cape Town who was also a doctor, so I phoned him and said, 'The doctors here won't pass me as A-1,' but he got me in as A-1. Today, I'll say the first doctor was right, because we had to walk in hot, deep sand and I found it very difficult!

"We were a volunteer group and the first white women in a military hospital to look after blacks in South Africa because their hospitals had only trained black men and doctors. To work there, we had to be between 25 and 30, mentally stable, and physically fit. Our unit had 30 nurses, 36 NCOs [Non Commissioned Officers], a number of doctors, and supposedly eight trained black orderlies but only two turned up. We went by boat to Egypt, and the nursing staff and doctors stayed outside Cairo while the NCOs built the hospital and put up our tents. The only permanent building on site was Matron's and the CO's [Commanding Officer's] office. The bathroom was built from clay and straw, and the toilet was a hole in the ground, and some distance from the bathroom, which had the showers, baths and washbasins. We walked from the toilet to the bathroom to get washed! We wore khaki uniforms with the South African emblem, and as I was a captain, I also had three pips on mine. We had a special hat, but on duty, we wore a white uniform with a veil, similar to that worn by English Sisters. After four and a half years, it ruined your hair! Our skin became very dehydrated and we had no way to get cream. It took a lot out of us and I think we looked 20 years older when we got out of that place.

"The hospital had space for 1200 patients and 200 of them had bacillary dysentery. I had two staff nurses, two orderlies, and some untrained orderlies on my floor. Patients could go to the bathroom if they were allowed up, but if not, we emptied bedpans in a hole in the ground and cleaned them with eusol. Sterilization was impossible! Conditions on the wards were very primitive and one nurse had a nervous breakdown after six months. There were flies, lice, and things that crawled, like scorpions. They were on the food everywhere, but there wasn't a thing you could do about it. We couldn't wear toeless shoes and always had to shake our shoes out; something I did for months after I came home!

"I worked in the infectious block with 350 patients, of whom 200 had VD. White orderlies looked after them and gave them M and B 693 which was the nearest thing we had to an antibiotic. When they came back with VD, we discovered that they put the pills in their pocket and sold them on the black market! Patients had meningitis, pneumonia, typhoid, typhus; we had everything! There was nothing we could do for meningitis, only sponge them to keep their temperatures down and give them aspirin. We put typhoid patients in cold water to bring the temperature down, which I think was as traumatic for them as it was for us! But they did feel better afterwards because it brought their temperature down.

"Our patients were isolated and we wore gowns and masks. We had a group of patients who were lonely and wanted to be with other patients from their village so they went down to the surgical ward after everybody was gone. When we did rounds the next morning, we found patients with mumps and chickenpox were next to patients who had appendix surgery. We had an orderly who spoke their language and told them to stay in their section. We did what we could, but how much can you do for people when you can't talk to them? We had a terrific job getting them straightened out!

"We did get two or three patients with leprosy but only because the recruiting officer made a mistake and missed their symptoms. I had one patient who was isolated when it was discovered he had leprosy. When he realized what he had, he went to the bathroom and cut his throat. We just watched him die because we had nothing to keep him alive, not even a suction machine. It was the most terrible experience of my life, not being able to help him. I stayed with him that night until he died the next morning. We had somebody who could speak his language, but he just wanted to die and made no effort.

"In 1942 a convoy came from West Africa with 25,000 black troops on board. When they arrived in Egypt, 10,000 of them were ill with mumps, chicken pox, or smallpox because they were crammed in boats that only held 15,000. We put them in tents at the base camp, sorted them out, took their temperatures, and the British doctors diagnosed them as best they could. We had 650 patients admitted within 24 hours. Among them were four smallpox cases, one so virulent that the patient only lived 24 hours.

A British doctor visited him, and although he had been inoculated, he was dead within ten days. Smallpox patients were kept far away from the hospital because they didn't want to expose any more people than necessary. I was Head Nurse of the infectious block so I took care of them. I was vaccinated five times in three weeks because it wouldn't take and they were petrified that something would happen to me. I didn't get smallpox but my foot dropped completely and was so swollen I had to go off duty. The CO decided he'd send me back to South Africa to be booted out of the army, but I decided otherwise. I said, 'What I'm doing is unnatural. It doesn't make sense. Put me on a medical ward with a hundred patients. I'll be okay and give me one month to recover.' He did, but only on my honour that I would go home if I weren't better. I took great care of it and at the end of the month, it had improved.

"I shared a tent for four and a half years with an Australian nurse who was head of the operating room. The OR was made of clay and straw with ventilation holes at the top. When we had sand storms, the sand would come in through these holes. You could do nothing but sew up the patients, sand and all! Smithy would get livid because she had no sterilizing facilities. She only had a primus stove and would put a basin on it with the things to be sterilized. But the stove would explode and soot would be over everything! She'd get so mad and tear off to the CO, but it was very difficult to work under those conditions

"I remember a sand storm we had on March 17, 1942, which lasted three days! A group of us were coming off duty, and it was a black dark so we couldn't see to get back for supper. My future husband (whom I didn't know then) was on duty in the administrative block and realized we couldn't get back, so he and another NCO came and got on either side of us and walked us to the mess for supper. One of the girls tried to get back on her own but blew up against the fence and broke her arm! We got to the mess and the cook was bringing over beef for thirty people when the wind blew it off into the desert and he came in with an empty plate! There was sand in our food for days and we were dirty until the storm blew over. Another night the sand storm cleared around ten o'clock, and Smithy and I were so sick of being dirty that we had a bath and shook out our tents, sheets and clothes. We weren't in bed an hour when it started again. We just covered up and went to sleep!

"The winters were cold and miserable, and temperatures dropped to about 30. I'd have five blankets, bed socks, flannelette pajamas, a balaclava cap on, and a hot water bottle in bed and my coat over all that. In the morning we walked to the toilet, then back to the tent, picked up the washcloth, and went in the other direction to the bathroom to wash before going on duty at seven o'clock. In the summer it was between 100 and 120 degrees in the shade, but after a couple of years we got used to it. We slept under mosquito nets, but we didn't have to when we did nights. The temperature in the tent was about 90 or 100 degrees, and it was very hot under the mosquito net but you went under it because of the sand flies and mosquitoes. We took quinine for malaria and injections for typhoid. I was one of the few people who went through that place without a day off duty.

"I felt safe with the natives for the first two years because they showed us a great deal of respect. I did night duty one month in ten and we were in a blackout because it was a war area. I did three rounds a night, spoke to the orderly in charge, and saw any sick patients. I did them alone with only a flashlight so I wouldn't fall over the guard ropes between the tents. After two years in Egypt we discovered there was no colour barrier and blacks were allowed to mix with Egyptian girls. The blacks started to take advantage of the situation and we became fearful of them. One of the nurses found a black native under her bed and that scared us. They put a ten-foot wall around the compound, with glass on the top, and had an armed guard at the gate 24 hours a day. When I did night duty after that, I had a white sergeant with me because it wasn't safe to do rounds alone. While you're in that situation, you accept it, but thinking about it afterwards, you wonder how you managed.

"My future husband, Laurie, joined the South African forces and when asked his occupation, said he had a flower nursery. When he got to Egypt he was assigned as a nurse to my section where we had bacillary dysentery! After two days, he said to the doctor, 'Get me out of here. I can't stand this place.' They put him in the administrative block and he was responsible for admissions and discharges. We had a terrific turnover of patients; I had as many as 45 discharges in one day. It was a terrible job keeping the bed count correct, but Laurie developed a system whereby we knew the ward and bed number, like ward 1, bed 1, and this is how we knew the patients. It was very impersonal but we couldn't pronounce their names. I had patients from the Belgian Congo, which is now Nigeria, who spoke some French, and I thought my Montreal French wasn't too bad until I tried it on them! I had 45 lined up to go to Laurie's office at eight o'clock. I called each of them by their regimental number and they all answered each time. I phoned Laurie and said, 'You better come up and get these patients or they won't be there at eight o'clock.' He came up and, with his Parisian French, had them lined up in about five minutes!

"We had blacks from all parts of Africa. Most were Swahili but some came from West Africa and could speak English. One of the doctors got a dictionary and we learned Swahili for the conditions we were nursing. I could ask how many bowel movements, if they had pain in their stomach, or a headache. Other than that we had no communication with them. They were soldiers and the army tried to get them up to the front line, but with the first bomb, they went into a hole. They built roads and mostly did labour, but when danger came, they scrambled.

"El Alamein was the last line of defence in North Africa, and when the war moved towards there we were close to the front. Rommel was moving across the desert and we didn't have much defence, but we had to stay where we were and hope for the best. When the battle of El Alamein began, we were told to expect the worst, that we could be taken as POWs. We were under the Geneva Convention and had a red cross on the hospital but no other defence. They decided that half the nurses would leave and half asked to volunteer to stay with the patients in case we were taken prisoner. Some nurses had family in South Africa, but there was no reason why I couldn't volunteer so I did.

"Fortunately Rommel lost. Montgomery stopped him dead, which ended the North African campaign. It was one of the greatest victories of the war really. There was a great deal of tension for the patients and all of us. I went deaf a week after the battle. Nobody knew what happened but they believed it was the tension. It didn't bother me but it did keep me from going to Italy with the other girls. I had to stay in Egypt because Matron thought if I went to Italy and we came near the front line again, my deafness and my foot would work against me. I stayed at the base camp until the war was over. After I got out of the army, I wore a hearing aid.

"Initially the social life was hectic because we were new and weren't tired. We had an Australian camp, a New Zealand camp, and a British Hospital close by and we got a lot of invitations. But there were only thirty nurses so we'd divide up and ten would go to each place. We'd go and come back together and usually have a dance and something to eat and drink. The men went to a lot of trouble because they liked to see people before they went back to the desert knowing some of them might never come back. Later, we didn't have time for a social life because we were just too tired!

"We got two weeks off every six months and we'd go to places like Palestine, Syria, Lebanon, and Alexandria. I crossed the Sinai

Desert to Palestine by car and came back on an Egyptian train. I went to Alexandria two or three times because I loved it. It was beautiful! We'd go as a group to Cairo or Ishmael by bus or hospital transport. You seldom went on your own. When I got to know my husband better, we'd go to Cairo for the day. We were there on VE Day and when we got back to camp, everybody was partying. We didn't know the war was over. There were a lot of celebrations that night! I was coming home from Egypt by boat on VJ Day when Japan surrendered.

"My husband was a Dutch bulb grower from Holland. We decided to marry after the war and got married in 1946 and stayed in Cape Town until 1947. I went to work in public health after I got married but gave it up after six weeks because I was too tired to work! The desert sunsets had been beautiful, but the heat, the tension, and the living conditions were too difficult. My husband wanted to go to Holland because his mother was ill and I said, 'If you go to Holland, I will go to see my family' because my father and sister had died while I was away. We went to Holland, then to Newfoundland. He loved it and wanted to stay, so we set up the Holland Nurseries on Torbay Road.

"Laurie and I received similar medals because we went through the same campaign. The Africa Service Medal was given to those who served in North Africa. The British Defense Medal was issued to all service people who served from 1939 to 1945, and the British also gave the 1939 to '45 Star to those who went through the North African Campaign. The fourth medal is a special one called 'Oh My Garter' to commemorate a visit to the North Africa forces by General Smutz's wife. We had miniatures made so we could wear them as ceremonial medals. I only wore mine once when we were invited to the opening of the university because Laurie was Dutch Consul for the province. After dinner, Dr. McPherson came over and said, 'Jennie, you must be the most medaled woman in the room!' I felt very proud; it was a tremendous honour to have them.

"I nursed from 1936 until 1946 and stopped after I got married. I went back nursing in 1963 when Laurie became ill and I had to work. I was thankful I had my profession. I did a refresher course and was asked to go into nursing education. I didn't want to teach but felt I had something to give students in the clinical area. I worked there until my foot cracked up, like it did in Egypt, from walking to and from the residence and clinical area. I was well into my 50s so I applied for a disability pension and worked in the School of Nursing library until I retired.

"Nursing made my life really and I can't imagine my life without having been a nurse. I enjoyed every minute of it! It's given me much more meaning and tremendous satisfaction to know I was able to help so many people. It helped me as a mother and as a wife. Nursing certainly has changed in the last 50 years. I'm glad I trained when I did and had time with the patients. It gave me a lot of satisfaction and that's something I'm very, very happy about."

CHAPTER 9:

Ethel Williams

*"They respected me. If they didn't,
I don't think I would have been nursing so long."*

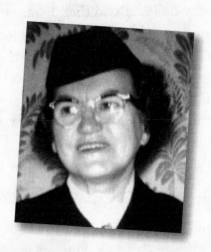

Ethel Williams [Williams] received the Order of Canada in 1984 because for forty years she served as a Public Health Nurse providing medical services to people living in isolated settlements around Placentia Bay. She delivered over 300 babies, extracted teeth, treated wounds, prescribed medication, and gave inoculations. (Source: *The Packet*)

Ethel Williams graduated from the Grace Hospital in 1935. "I entered in 1931, and was in six months before I got my cap. A couple of weeks later, I had to go home because my mother was ill. I brought her to see Dr. Roberts in St. John's, but he told me there was nothing he could do for her, so I took her home. Major Fagner gave me leave to look after her until she died. While I was home I didn't think I'd take up nursing again because I felt so downhearted, but around Christmas I got a message from Major Fagner to report for duty. I asked my brother what to do and he thought I should go back, so I went back in 1932.

"Nursing was important to me because when I was a little girl, my mother had an operation at the old General and she told me the different things they did at the hospital. I used a little plastic pan to make a bedpan for my doll and said then I was going to be a nurse. When I finished high school I still wanted to go into nursing.

"I worked in the post office for a year after I finished school. I wanted to go into nursing when I was eighteen but I didn't get in until I was twenty. I wanted to go to the General where my mother had been a patient, but I applied to General and the Grace and the Grace accepted me. My mother made all my uniforms. It was a joy for her to know I was going into nursing. The hardest part was that she wasn't there to see it all. If I had my life to live over again I would do the same thing!

"In the beginning we were called 'probies' and one of our duties was to scrub the walls of the operating room, clean all the instruments, the floors, and the bathroom. First when I went in training, two of us were sent to the bathroom to clean the bedpans. We scoured them with Ajax, shined them, and then took them to the basement to be sterilized. We did this every week. I had six piled up on my arm and the other girl had six. As we going downstairs two doctors were coming up so we took our aprons and put them over the bedpans so the doctors couldn't see them. I was so ashamed, going with those bedpans! It was funny, but we got caught using our aprons that way and lost a late leave.

"When we did nights we were supposed to go to bed as soon as you got off at 8 a.m., but one morning three of us decided to go downtown. About ten o'clock, we were dressed and ready to go when we heard a couple of supervisors checking to see if we were in bed. The three of us jumped in bed, boots and all on, and covered up to our necks. When they came into the room, I heard the Head Nurse say, 'Shh! They're sleeping. Don't wake them.' They closed the door and went. After about ten minutes we figured they were gone, so we got up and went downtown. We got back about one or two o'clock, went to bed, and had a nap!

"Every morning we had to be up, washed, dressed and report to prayers at six o'clock. One morning several of us were so tired we decided not to go to prayers. We slept in, thinking nobody would notice, but the next thing we knew the three of us were called to the office and asked why we didn't report for prayers. We said we were tired but we lost our leave and that morning we weren't allowed to go to coffee break. By twelve o'clock we were just about starved and one of the girls who belonged to St. John's phoned her parents who sneaked a lunch into us. We ate it in the bathroom!

"In my last year of training I was on nights for six months and spent them in the OR. It was too long but I enjoyed it. We had fun, which was the only thing that got us through. We assisted the doctors with appendectomies and other operations. I definitely liked the OR, but I also liked the delivery room. I assisted with about 25 deliveries, including a set of triplets. When the lady came in, she said she was having a twin but she had no doctor. I said, 'Miss Thomas, please let me deliver the babies,' and she did! The woman had two boys and a girl, and they were all perfect. Two were five pounds and the other one was six. The woman was huge but her babies were healthy!

"I had my first brush with death in training. I was bringing blood work to the lab late one evening and as I went through the corridor I was faced with this corpse, the first one I ever saw. Her face wasn't covered up and she was lying there like somebody asleep. It gave me such a scare! I returned to the floor, frightened stiff because I thought the corpse was after me. Back on the ward I told one of the nurses what happened and she said, 'Come on. I'll go with you.' The nurse came with me and I touched the corpse, which helped me get over it. They had put the corpse near the lab, waiting to go into the morgue.

"My next experience with death was an eight-year-old boy who died from appendicitis. I got him ready after death because there were no funeral homes then, so we did them up in the hospital. I washed him and put on his clothes but every time I moved him he'd grunt. You wouldn't know but he was speaking to you! It gave me a funny feeling but I didn't mind it."

Ethel returned to Woody Island after graduation but it was two years before she began working in public health. In the interim she delivered babies and encountered superstitions and old wives' tales surrounding health practices on the island. She also encountered some unusual methods of delivering babies.

"When I went to Woody Island first, I was on my own. Wireless was the only connection I had with Come By Chance hospital. I had to write the Director of Nurses if I wanted to know anything, and I couldn't get a doctor without wiring for him. It took a couple of hours unless it was an emergency and then it went above everything else. The roads on the island were so slippery, and I put socks over my boots and they would stick to the ice. I don't know how many pairs I wore out! My dad made creepers out of galvanized spikes to put on my boots, and only for him, I would have been killed. I had an accident about ten years ago and the doctor said to me, 'I believed you had ribs broken before.' I said, 'I probably did and didn't do anything about it.' I never had time to look after myself and I couldn't be bothered going to the doctor for every ache or pain.

"Growing up on Woody Island, we were never told anything. I remember my cousin and me trying to raise a huge rock with two long sticks because we were told that's where the babies were and we intended to get one. We never found the baby and were very disappointed!

"Once I had a nosebleed in school and really bled. First they treated me by hanging cold keys around my neck. Then they put rocks around my neck. I was walking home from school with my friend and she kept saying, 'Are you all right?' because rocks were dropping from me. Finally when I got home they put ice packs on my nose which stopped the bleeding. When I was about eleven, the midwife on Woody Island was told about my nosebleeds and she said she could cure them. She came to our house and tied a piece of green ribbon around my neck. She called it charmed! She said, 'Don't take it off. Leave it on until it falls off.' It must have been on for two years and rotted off my neck, but I never had any nosebleeds since. I don't know how it worked!

"I had 35 warts on my hand before I went in training and I said to my mother, 'What am I going to do about them?' She said, 'We'll get Aunt Dora because she charmed your nosebleeds and will take away your warts.' Aunt Dora came and counted every wart. That was all I thought of it but the warts went away. Later, Aunt Dora told me what she did: 'I counted your warts and marked out 35 strokes with chalk on the back of the stove and said, "In the name of the Father, Son and Holy Ghost" for each one. That's how your warts went.' I never had any since so there must be something to it!

"The people on Woody Island knew I was a nurse and wanted me to deliver their baby. Up to that time, there were two midwives who would go together. Midwifery knowledge was handed from one midwife to the other. They knew how to cut the cord but I don't think they knew much about cleanliness. They never wore rubber gloves but they probably washed their hands. The midwife would always say, 'You're in the family way.' My sister-in-law was expecting her third baby and I said, 'I'll deliver your baby seeing as I'm home.' People didn't know what pregnant was and my aunt came to the house one day and said, 'What's wrong with R?' I said, 'She's pregnant and I'm going to deliver her baby.' Well, that news went around the island to all seventy-five families. One day the midwife came to the house and said, 'R. is pregent, is she?' I said, 'What?' She said, 'I heard she was pregent.' She didn't know the word was pregnant! She called it pregent!

"I had a patient who I knew was going to have a difficult labour, in fact she had a caesarian delivery, and her family was very illiterate. I took her to the doctor and while he was registering her, he said, 'You're pregnant, aren't you?' 'No sir!' she said, 'I'm Church of England.' She didn't know what pregnant was! We nearly passed out and I had to walk away!

"I was called to deliver a woman who was progressing well and I was having supper with her husband while I was waiting for her to be ready to deliver. He said, 'Nurse, make sure you bring along a boy because we don't want any girls in this house.' I said, 'What can I do to arrange for a boy, I wonder?' Anyway, their rooster jumped up on the fence and crowed. The man looked at me and said, 'Do you know what that rooster said?' I said, 'It said it's a girl.' He said, 'If I thought he said it's a girl I'd chop the head off that bird!' By then the patient was calling out to me, and in 15 minutes, the baby was born. It was a girl! I didn't know what to do! When I came out, the husband asked me, 'What is it?' I said, 'It's a girl.' He said, 'Don't tell me you brought along a girl,' and then he said to his wife, 'Give me the axe and I'll chop the head off the rooster.' He did kill it later. They had a son who died and he wanted another boy.

"One of my patients was having her seventh baby and was in labour about 24 hours. I got worried because labour shouldn't last that long and I wondered what I was going to do. There was no doctor but we did have telephone connections between Woody Island and Come by Chance. You rang Garden Cove and they connected you to the hospital. I couldn't leave the patient so I wrote my husband Beaton a note, told him what the patient was like and said, 'Get Dr. Coxen on the line and tell him I'm in difficulty. I can't get the baby to deliver.' The doctor said, 'Put a binder around her abdomen and as the baby is coming down, tie it tighter and keep it tight. Each time the patient has a pain and the baby is coming down, tie it a bit tighter until you drive the baby out.' I did and it worked. I had no problems but I never had to use the procedure again. The baby was perfect, a 13-pound boy. Practically a grown man!

"One Sunday morning I was getting ready for church when two men came to the door from Monkstown. One man said, 'My little girl is sick and I'd like you to see her.' I said to him, 'Okay,' and to the other man, 'What's your trouble?' He said, 'It's my niece. She had her baby but can't finish the work and they want you to come.' We had to go to Clattice Harbour in a boat, which was a three-hour run from Woody Island. Then we had to walk 25 minutes and finally go 14 miles by motorboat to Monkstown. I said, 'We can go into Bar Haven on the way down and see how the little girl is,' but she only had a slight cold. We went on to Monkstown and when I walked into the patient's room, her legs were tied above the knee with rags and her arms were tied across her abdomen. I said to the midwife, 'Why have you got her tied up? Is she going crazy?' She said, 'To keep her from bleeding.' I said, 'Help me untie her quickly.' When we untied her, I put my hand on her abdomen over the placenta and had no trouble at all. She did bleed a lot but I got it under control. I met up with this kind of practice all the time. I stayed with the patient until eleven o'clock that night. I told them what to do and to telephone if they needed me. I had to go home the way I came but they wouldn't let me go down the bay because I was too tired. A lady in Clattice Harbour made me a cup of tea and said, 'Get up to bed.' She had a hot water bottle in the bed for me and I appreciated that more than anything. I didn't wake until nine the next day and got home about noon.

"On Fools' Day, April 1, the maid of the woman next door came up and said, 'Mrs. J. would like you to come down. She thinks her baby is going to be born.' I didn't think it would arrive for another 10 or 12 days so I said, 'This is Fools' Day. Go back and tell her, I'm not coming down because she's not expecting her baby yet.' I thought, 'They're trying to fool me.' She came up later and said, 'Mrs. J said to come down, she wants you.' I took my bag but when I got on the bridge, Beaton's brother was there and he said, 'Where are you going?' I said, 'Next door, she's expecting her baby.' He said, 'I was just there and everything is fine. It's Fools' Day, my dear, they're having a bit of fun with you. Go home.' I went back to the house and the girl came back again with a note from Mrs. J: 'This is no Fools' Day, come as quickly as possible.' The note was all I needed. I took my bag and went. My brother-in-law was in the door laughing at me and I said, 'This is no Fools' Day trick!' I was only there half an hour when the baby was delivered.

"I delivered over 300 babies and only one died. That was my last year on Woody Island because we moved to Arnold's Cove with the resettlement program. The family had the midwife but called me when there was trouble. I knew the mother couldn't deliver, so I contacted Dr. Coxen, who came and delivered the baby, but mother and baby died. He was there in plenty of time but couldn't do a thing to help!

"First when I started with public health, I would go to the

outports to do clinics and visit schools. I'd go on the coastal boat and be gone about two days before coming back. One time I had no boarding house and didn't know where to stay so I asked the post mistress where I could stay for the night. She said, 'You can stay with me but you'll have to sleep in the priest's room because it's the only room I've got.' I said, 'I don't mind where it is, anywhere will do me.' When it came time to go to bed, she showed me the room, which was off the kitchen. It had no curtain or blind on the window, and the road passed right next to that window. I had a flashlight and the room had a kerosene oil lamp. I thought, 'I can't have the light on because anybody going along the road will see me,' so I blew the lamp out and used my flashlight. I was very tired because I had worked hard that day so I got in the bed, fell back on the pillow, and struck the back of my head with something. I thought, 'I'm killed!' I was afraid to pull back the pillow thinking there might be a gun under it, but when I did, it was an unopened bottle of rum. I wondered what I was going to do with it, take it home for Christmas or tell the lady about it. I thought maybe the priest put it there and forgot it. Anyway I could hear the lady going up and down the stairs and stopping by my room. She did this three or four times so I called out to her to come in. She came in and I said, 'Look what I found under the pillow.' 'Oh, my dear,' she said, 'I hid that from my husband because he was drinking all day and I was sure he was going to drink it. He's as blind as a bat and I thought the priest's bed was a very good place to put it.' I said, 'Well, you nearly knocked my head off!' She said, 'I'm really sorry!' I gave her the bottle of rum and didn't have it for Christmas.

"My district included Woody Island, Bar Haven, Davis Cove, Monkstown, and sometimes Clattice Harbour. Often I was on the wharf getting ready to get aboard the boat to make my visits when Beaton would be coming home from work with the Department of Highways. Other times, I'd be stepping back on the wharf and he'd be boarding the boat to go back to work in Swift Current. It was the way life went for us for 38 years but I enjoyed every moment. We had a wonderful marriage, with one daughter, and I'd do the same thing all over again if I had to.

"The people on Woody Island really relied on me. I always had a flag and when I arrived home, my flag would go up to let the people know I was back, and when I'd leave, the flag was lowered. I used it all the time and it was a good signal to the community. Mr. Williams had the store on the island and he always knew where I was. That was a big help.

"Once a month the ship, *Lady Anderson*, went to Rushoon, Petite Forte, and Fortune Bay. She'd also go around Placentia Bay and occasionally come into Woody Island. It was a government boat that came around in the summer. Doctor Coxen was on the *Lady Anderson* and if I asked him to see a patient, he'd grab his bag and come. The people thought the *Lady Anderson* was great because with a doctor on board they thought they had it made. I got a message one day to go to Davis Cove to see a woman in labour, and the *Lady Anderson* was at Woody Island which was about one and a half miles from my clinic. I went to the boat and asked the captain to take me to Davis Cove. I said, 'Maybe the doctor on board would like to come along to deliver the baby.' The doctor came out of his room and wanted to know what was going on and when I told him, he said, 'We'll take you but I'm not having anything to do with the patient.' It took us about an hour and a half to get there and as I was getting off I said to the doctor, 'Aren't you coming with me? What if there are complications? It would be nice to have you there.' He said, 'I'm not coming with you,' then looked at the captain and said, 'Take off, we're not staying here.' With that the captain let go the lines and I was left alone with the patient. He was a Dr. W from somewhere in England. I met the captain sometime later and he apologized for leaving me.

He said, 'I wanted to come back but the doctor said no.' I think the doctor was vexed because I got the call and he didn't, but the patient didn't know the boat was at Woody Island so she wired me. Sometimes you ran into jealousy like that from some of the doctors.

"Tuberculosis [TB] was rampant and Beaton had three sisters with TB; two died at home and his third sister was burnt to death in a boarding house in St. John's while she was waiting for a bed at the San. The people on Woody Island claimed it [TB] was caused by the hooked rugs they used on their floors. When I came home from the Grace Hospital my sister-in-law had four or five on her kitchen floor and we got rid of them because she had two small children and people would come who weren't very careful about spitting. They'd smoke the pipe or chew tobacco and didn't mind spitting on the floor. I had my hands full, teaching people about spitting. My tongue never ceased! They'd tell me I was stuck up and thought I knew it all because I had been in training. They believed me, though, because I did see an improvement. They respected me because if they didn't, I don't think I would have been nursing so long.

"I had to lay out people for burial. The nurse did it because nobody else would touch them. It was no good for me to say, 'Get somebody else to do it because I have other work to do.' Sometimes, a next-door neighbour might come in to help, but she was afraid to touch them so I had to do it all myself. They'd get the casket ready, which they built themselves. I'd wash the body, pack it, and put on whatever clothes they had. The jaws were tied up with a bandage. They had what was called a winding sheet, which was three or four yards of shirting with notches cut out and little trimmings around the edges. You doubled up the shirting and when you cut it, it had a diamond shape. You'd put this in the casket and roll the patient in it. It was the tradition at the time. The worst thing about getting the body ready was when you turned it over, the air in their lungs escaped, giving you a good fright! I'd think they were going to talk to me. It was an awful feeling!

"One year I delivered two babies on the day before Christmas Eve and was called out at two o'clock that night to deliver another one. I came home Christmas morning and was so tired! My husband said, 'Now, Ethel, you're going to bed after breakfast and this is one day you're not going anywhere. I'll cook dinner and call you around eleven o'clock. This is it! I'm laying down the law!' And he really meant business! As we were eating breakfast, I said, 'Beaton, two men are coming over the hill. I wonder what they want.' He said, 'Don't forget what I told you!' I went to the door and the man said, 'I'm sorry, Nurse, to come for you on Christmas Day but my wife is dying.' What could I do! I asked him into the kitchen and said, 'Beaton, this man came from Bar Haven, his wife is dying. What am I going to do?' Beaten got up from the table and said, 'When duty calls her danger, be never wanting there. Pack your bag and go!' Best words I ever heard! I went to the clinic in the basement, got my bag, and left for Bar Haven. I delivered the baby and everything was fine. I had my Christmas dinner in Bar Haven, and about three o'clock that afternoon I decided to go visiting because the patient was okay. As I was walking up the road I noticed a motorboat coming in the harbour and it looked like a Woody Island boat. It was my husband with his brother and a couple of other people, who came to Bar Haven to see how I was getting on. I went to meet them and Beaton said, 'We have lots of time so we'll stay here. It's Christmas day.' I went back to see my patient who was okay. Then we had supper on the other side of the harbour with friends and went home that night. We had a lovely Christmas Day!"

As a Public Health Nurse, Ethel Williams was the only health professional in the area and made herself available to the people when they needed her. However, there were those who could take advantage of her presence under somewhat questionable circumstances.

"They wired me from Monkstown and told me to go to Davis Cove. I walked eight miles with three men and over four ponds to get there and the road was bad. I thought it must be a very sick person I was going to see. When I got there everything was normal and I couldn't find a thing wrong with her. I questioned her and sometimes she would talk to me and other times she wouldn't. I figured she must be mental. I got her a cup of coffee and talked to her and got her smiling a bit. I couldn't go back home that night, and I was really tired so I stayed at the boarding house in Monkstown. The people there said, 'There's nothing wrong with that one. We know her, she's just shamming.' I said, 'If I thought I walked eight miles for someone shamming, I don't know what I would do with her because I'm so tired I'm ready to drop!' I went back to see her in the morning and she was fine, not a thing wrong with her! I had to walk eight miles to get home and when I got back my legs gave out and I could hardly walk across my kitchen. I later found out she had stolen money from her brother. He worked away and saved $2000 to get a house because he was getting married, and she took the money. That was her trouble!

"We had only one maternity patient on Woody Island this particular night and about two o'clock in the morning a rap came on the door. I got up and opened my bedroom window, which was over the front door, and asked a couple of times who was there but nobody spoke. My daughter Betty heard it and called out that someone had knocked. I told her I thought it might be the lady who was pregnant and that I was going up to see if she was okay. My daughter said, 'You're not going out on a night like this alone.' I said, 'I'll be all right, you watch me through the window,' because it wasn't a dark night. There was nobody around when I came down so I got my bag and went up the road. About halfway up, I looked down the garden and thought I saw a ghost. A man was standing in the garden waving his hands at me and I really thought it was a ghost. I was frightened so I turned around and went home. When I got in the house, Betty said, 'Mom, what happened?' I said, 'Not much, but I don't think I'll go up now.' I couldn't tell her! She said, 'I'll go up with you.' We had electricity at Woody Island then and I had heard that if you saw a ghost and turned on the light, the bulb would burst. I turned on the light and it didn't go out! I thought, 'There's no ghost so I'll go back again.' I told Betty to go back to bed and went up to the house. As I passed the garden, I took a good look and it was only a tree with the branches fluking [moving rapidly, twitching] back and forth just like hands waving to me! As I climbed the hill to get to the house, I slipped and fell several times, but finally made it. When I went into the kitchen, a man was in the rocking chair and I said, 'Did you come for me, sir?' 'Yes,' he said. His wife was in the next room and I didn't have time to wash my hands or do anything. I hauled on my rubber gloves, grabbed my plastic apron, put it on and delivered the baby. That's how much time I had! I was still wearing my cap and coat! When I finished up I asked the man why he didn't wait for me. 'I had an awful time trying to get here.' But he just rocked back and forth and didn't mind me one bit. I said, 'You'll wait for me the next time,' and he said, 'There'll be no next time, Nurse.' I delivered three more babies for him after that and he waited for me! Some people didn't have any regard for what the nurse went through.

"I had a similar case on the lower part of Woody Island. I lived in the middle cove of Woody Island. About two or three o'clock one morning a man came for me, then he left! The teacher on Woody Island was boarding with me and he heard me getting ready and called out, 'Nurse, did that man go off without you?' I said, 'Yes,' and he said, 'I'll go with you.' We had to go over three hills covered with ice and snow. Only for him I would have been killed because I couldn't get there myself. When I got to the house, here was the man sitting in his chair! The teacher spent the night at a friend's house and waited until I was ready to go home ten o'clock the next morning.

"I held my clinics in one community and everyone would come from around the area to get their children inoculated. This day I was vaccinating 85 children. I ate my breakfast eight o'clock that morning and by two o'clock, I was hungry! The boarding mistress had come into the room several times and finally she said, 'Nurse, if you don't have something to eat I'm going to send the people home.' I asked one of the patients who was very reliable if she would look after things until I got back so I could have a cup a tea. As I was going into the kitchen, this 75-year-old lady said, 'Where you going, Nurse?' I said, 'I'm going to get a cup of tea.' She said, 'What's a big thing like you want with something to eat. For goodness sake, girl, go back to work. You don't want anything to eat.' I said, 'I'm having something to eat and I don't think that you're that sick that you can't wait a few minutes longer.' She said, 'There's nothing wrong with me, I got arthritis, that's all.' You met up with this sort of thing lots of times.

"One evening about six o'clock, just before the post office closed, I got a telegram saying 'Come immediately, very ill.' When I got there, the patient was on the wharf to meet me, so I said to her, 'I got your message and thought you were sick but it must be somebody else in the house.' 'Oh no,' she said, 'I'm the sick one.' She was 44 and in menopause; that's all was wrong with her! I talked to her and gave her a 222 tablet because she was having a lot of pain, but I had to stay in a boarding house for the night.

"I was only home for a couple hours when I got another message from Monkstown. They would bring the patient to Davis Cove so I could see her there. Beaton was home so he took me in the boat. We waited at Davis Cove for an hour for them to come with the patient on a horse and sleigh. It was a little boy about nine and his mother. The poor horse was just about dead from hauling her, the boy, and her husband eight miles; it took two to three hours. The mother said, 'Nurse, he's got a broken collarbone.' I said, 'Did he fall down?' She said, 'No, but it's broken. I can feel it.' I felt around but couldn't feel anything abnormal so I said, 'His collarbone isn't broken.' The youngster spoke up, 'That's not what's wrong, Mom, it's my tooth!' I said, 'What's wrong with your tooth?' He opened his mouth and I said, 'It looks like a gum boil. You have an infected tooth.' He didn't have a temperature but I gave him some tablets and told him, 'They will clear it up in no time.' I said to the mother, 'Stay in Davis Cove tonight and go back in the morning.' 'No,' she said, 'I wanted to go down the bay and I've got my suitcases packed to go. If you don't let us go down, we're going home.' I said, 'Why did you want to go down the bay?' She said, 'That's where I want to go.' I said, 'My dear, you won't be going down no bay with me tonight. If you're not staying in Davis Cove, take the boy home so he can get his night's sleep. I'll be visiting the school in Davis Cove in a couple days and I want to see the boy then.' She pretended he had a broken collarbone and had me travel three hours by boat, then expected me to take her back with me. That was the sort of thing you had to put up with!

"One night I went to visit a patient about 2 a.m. and had to walk over the stage head rails. The boat captain said, 'I'm not letting you go up there alone. Give me your bag and I'll go with you.' When I got to the top there was no floor on the wharf. If I had taken a couple more steps I would have gone down on the rocks and been killed. Some 14- to 15-year-old boys had done it, I found out afterwards. I spoke to the Mounties about it afterwards and they said I should have notified them sooner. I said, 'No, it was their first time doing something like this so I forgave them. They were playing a trick on me but it was a very poor one!'

"When the Salk polio vaccine came out I gave the first injections in Davis Cove. You gave the first injection, waited a month, gave the second one, and after another month gave the third one. I went back to give approximately 70 school children and babies the second injection. When I arrived at the wharf an old gentleman asked me where I was going. I said, 'I'm going up to the school to give them their second injection.' He said, 'Don't go to the school because they're going to kill you. They all had swollen arms.' I kept going but the boat captain heard the old gentleman and said, 'Don't go.' But I was going. The captain got off the boat and came along behind me. I had to walk around the harbour about half a mile and met a couple of women who said, 'You're going to be killed today,' and asked me not to go. I said, 'This is my work and I'm going. I'm ready for it.' They all stared at me and were so frightened but I went on. I saw the captain was following me so I felt good about that. I rapped on the school door and the teacher came out and he looked frightened. He said, 'Nurse, you got some nerve coming here today.' I said, 'What's the trouble?' He said, 'I got 13- and 14-year-old pupils here and they're going to kill you.' I said, 'I don't think they're as bad as that. You tell them I'm here to give them their second injection, but if they don't want it, I'll go home and there'll be no more to it than that.' He said, 'I'll gladly do that.' I waited and I was some frightened! I could see the captain hidden behind bushes, watching. The teacher came out and said, 'Come on in.' When I went into the school, this big bully of a fellow stood up and said, 'What are you here for, Nurse?' I said, 'I'm back to give you the second needle because it is no good unless you have all three done. But that's up to you all. If you want it, okay, and if you don't I'll take my bag and leave. No more to it than that!' He stopped and all eyes were on me. 'Okay,' he said, 'come in. We'll have the needle.' I did them all and the mothers came with their babies. I never had a hitch after that!"

Despite the occasional misadventure, the people of Woody Island appreciated the work Ethel did and made every effort to support her. Many of her challenges in delivering health care resulted from the fact that the people were isolated and likely had unrealistic expectations of her role. "Father C. was the priest in Bar Haven and he was very nice. He made sure the person was sick before they came for me, and I appreciated that very much because if I got a call to go to Bar Haven, it took me nearly three hours to walk there. In winter, it would be blowing and drifting over the ponds and I'd have a man on each side of me. You couldn't walk across, you just ran because the wind would be at your back.

"If there was a storm some men would go with me and protect me from the drifts and guide me along the road. They'd put something like a shawl over my face and I'd have my shawl around my neck. I was out so many times when you couldn't see a hand before your face, and I would have to sit down in the snow to get my leg out of a drift. Woody Island and Bar Haven were bad places for snow drifts. How I ever got along, I don't know!

"Dr. Coxen taught me to extract teeth and I never had any problems. I had to suture and I remember an elderly man came to me because he had cut his leg in the woods. When I saw the cut, I said, 'I'm sending you to Come By Chance because the tendons might be cut.' 'Look here,' he said, 'if you don't sew up my leg, I'll get a needle and thread and do it myself. I'm not going to any hospital!' I said, 'Okay, but you'll have to take the consequences.' He was drunk and when I had six sutures in, I told the girl to get Beaton. He came up and said, 'Go ahead, sew it up now because he's as drunk as a fool and doesn't need anything to put him to sleep.' I put twelve sutures in him. Then we slapped cold water on his face, shook him, and got him up. He said, 'Got it finished?' And I said, 'Yes, but when the *Lady Anderson* comes around, I want you to go see the doctor on board and see if I've done it right.' He did go and the doctor told him he couldn't have done a better job himself. It was perfect!

"One day a man came in with a stick of wood stuck so far in his forefinger that I couldn't get at it and I wondered what I was going to do. I put a packed compress on it, told him to go home and put another compress on in about two hours and keep it on. Then come back on Sunday. The compress drew the splinter out enough that I could get it with the forceps. I pulled it out and put it in the stove. There wasn't that much to it. He thanked me and left. He met my husband's brother and said, 'Boy, that was some bad! The splinter was so big the nurse stumbled going to the stove to burn it.' That was the kind of thing they'd say. Could they ever exaggerate!

"A man came to the clinic complaining there was something wrong with his back passage. I said, 'You've probably got hemorrhoids.' 'What's that?' he said. I got him up on the examining table and did he ever have hemorrhoids. I said, 'I think I'll send you to the doctor.' So I wrote a note to the doctor in Come By Chance. Now this man and his wife couldn't read. The doctor gave him glycerin suppositories and thought no more about it. He told the man to come back in two weeks if he wasn't better, and when two weeks were up, the patient came to see me. I said, 'You have to go to the doctor in Come By Chance. So he went and bumped into the doctor in the corridor who asked him how he was getting on. 'Not very good,' he said. 'It would have been better if I had shoved those things you give me up my ass for what good they did me.' The doctor said, 'That's where I meant for you to put them. What did you do?' The man said, 'I ate them!' He had eaten three suppositories, got sick, and threw up! If he had come to me after he saw the doctor, I could have told him how to use them. The doctor told me afterwards that he thought the man could read the instructions on the box. But in those days many people couldn't read. The teacher on Woody Island had about 30 adults in school at night, teaching them to read and write. By the time she left, some could write their name. I don't know how they got along!

"One time when Beaton was in the woods, I spent the night with my sister-in-law. I told people where I would be if they wanted me. About ten o'clock, a man came to the house and said, 'My wife is having her baby. I think you better stay with us tonight.' We had to walk a mile and a half to his house and it was icy and very slippery. They had seven boys and he said, 'This time we want you to bring along a girl.' I said, 'I probably will bring along a girl.' He was carrying my bag and he slipped and lost it down the brook and out on the saltwater ice. I was scared because everything I needed was in that bag. I said, 'The bag is gone, and there's no girl for you tonight.' I waited on the road until he got the bag and when he came back with it, I looked at it and said, 'My son, it's a boy!' He said, "Nurse, if I thought it was a boy I'd leave you right where you are.' We went on and I was there two days before the baby came and it was another boy. When I came down to the kitchen, the husband was sitting by the fire. He said, 'What have you got for us this time?' I said, 'A boy.' 'My God!' he said. 'Take it, we don't want it.' Their last child was a daughter but I didn't deliver her. They wouldn't have me. My aunt was a trained midwife by then. She did a six-week course at the Grace and she got the girl for him!

"Nurse W. trained at the old General but came to the Grace for maternity. One night we had a patient who was not dilated and this nurse said to me, 'There's a little verse I'm going to repeat for you:

'Oh Lord, when we lay down our caps and cross the bar
Wilt Thou give us just one little star
To wear in our cap and a uniform new
In the city above, where the Head Nurse is You.'

"I never forgot that and have thought about it often. I must have been strong to do what I did. Sometimes I lie in bed wondering how I got through it all. I always felt there was somebody else there helping me. I couldn't do it myself. I suppose it was a good way to be.

"Nursing is physically strenuous. I had to climb over wharves, travel on horse and sled, and ski-doo, and that was hard on my back. That's where the hard work was but it wasn't easy delivering babies either. It was hard on the old head too with your brain working all the time. I really did enjoy nursing. I only wish that I were able to go back and do it all over again. I'd know more about it now."

CHAPTER 10:

Cluda Grandy

"You can't become familiar with people (staff).
How could I go in the dining room and not talk to them?
You had to sort of stand off. You couldn't help it. It wasn't that
I wished to be that way. I was expected to be dignified."

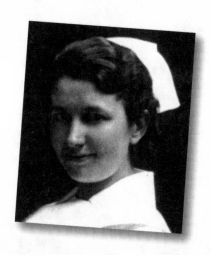

Following completion of the Maternity Program at the Grace
Hospital, Cluda Grandy worked at the Grand Bank Cottage
Hospital before returning to complete the general nursing
program. She spent most of her career in tuberculosis nursing,

first traveling with the mobile x-ray unit and finally as Director of Nursing at the Sanatorium in Corner Brook. She describes nursing as a lonely existence because she believed that being in charge prevented her from becoming 'familiar' with other nurses.

Cluda Grandy completed the one and a half year Maternity Nursing Program at the Grace Hospital. She was invited to work at the Grand Bank Cottage Hospital and remained there for three years before deciding she wanted to finish "training." In 1934 she entered the General Nursing Program at the Grace and graduated in 1935.

"In Grand Bank I was the Nurse-in-charge and I had two nursing assistants that I trained myself. They made beds and did baths and I did the medications and everything else. We didn't have night staff but each patient had a bell which was connected to my bedroom, and if they needed me they just rang. I'd get up and attend to them in my dressing gown. That wasn't very nice but there was no set time; you worked from when you got up until you went to bed at night. I had my own living room and was quite comfortable.

"It was a lonely life. I didn't see my family often because it was about 30 miles from Garnish to Grand Bank and they didn't have a car or a carriage. I got a two-week vacation but they'd have to get someone to replace me. I was United Church and I helped out with church activities whenever I could. If there was a special occasion and I could get away, I'd help out and the housekeeper would answer the bells because most of the time the patients would only want a drink or something like that. I didn't have time for boyfriends but I did make friends with a number of people from the church who invited me out. But I was the person responsible so I couldn't be gone very long from the hospital, and the housekeeper always covered while I was gone. I didn't really miss spending time with friends because if I stayed in to listen for patients, I'd read or listen to the radio. I'd get books from anywhere and there were a few books in the building for anyone that wanted them. I did a lot of fancy embroidery like luncheon cloths and I knit baby sweaters and booties and gave them away. I found it a lonely existence but the community did look up to me, although I didn't have much fun in Grand Bank.

"I did miss having another nurse with me there because I had no one to talk things over with. The doctor did make visits, sometimes twice a day, and I'd make rounds with him and talk things over with him then. Dr B. was the doctor and he was really concerned about the patients. He and his wife invited me to their home several times and I went when I could. They were good to me.

"The tidal wave happened in 1929 while I was working in Grand Bank. The place shook and we thought the furnace had blown up but it was over in a short time. I remember it because my grandmother belonged to Lamaline and that's why I was so interested in it, but she had died long before it happened. People were washed out to sea and homes floated out because the waves were so high the houses tumbled over. One house was going out to sea with the lamps still on. It was terrible! People drowned and there was no way to rescue them because the boats had been swept out with the wave. That was the worst part of it! I didn't know about all the damage that had been done in Lamaline because there were no cars and no one visited. In Newfoundland, the people built near the water because it was easier for the fishermen to get to their boats and that was why the homes were swept out. It was terrible and everyone was so upset over it. We didn't get any patients from St. Lawrence because they had their own nurse and she took care of them. Nurse C. was English and she lived further in from the beach so she wasn't affected by the wave. She used to come visit me and I had an extra bed for anyone like that."

After three years in Grand Bank, Cluda decided to return to the Grace Hospital to finish nursing. "I applied and told the doctor I was going back, and he thought it was a good idea and helped me with my application. I wanted to do nursing all my life because as a child I was always nursing my dolls.

"I spent a few weeks in Garnish with my people to let them know I was going back and to find out how they felt about it. They were delighted. My father was a boat builder and had a tinsmith business where he made things like pots and pans. They called it a tin factory. He used big sheets of tin and we made things from the pieces left over but we weren't allowed to touch the expensive stuff. It was small but it brought in money to bring up the family. Remember this was the '30s and things were difficult! We were fortunate because my father worked every day except Sundays. He was a wonderful person!

"I stayed at the Grace Hospital residence. It was nice because our room was at the top of the hospital and we could see out the windows. I thought it was a large room, but I've been back since and it wasn't as I remembered it. It had shrunk! I found it lonely in residence. I got to know the M.H. family in St. John's and they invited me out often. They lived up from the hospital, near St. Clare's. They were good to me and nice company. Gradually I got to know other people and it wasn't too bad at all. I had never used a phone but my family didn't have a phone so there was no way I could talk to them. Only rich people had a phone!

"The school liked the students to go to church when they had time and we got four hours off on Sunday to go. I never missed church but one night I was so tired I stayed home. I was in my bed and the door opened and in came Miss W. She said, 'I'm surprised at you, you a Christian, and here you are laughing and carrying on with the rest of them.' I wasn't carrying on but I felt so terrible! If my mother ever found out, she'd have a fit because my parents were very strict about church. I never heard anymore about it and I wasn't penalized but I didn't miss church again unless I was doing night duty. They were strict but fair.

"We got one day off in the week and some of us didn't even get that, just time off on Sundays. We didn't have much free time because we worked 12-hour days. We had to go out for games or things like that, so we'd just get together in the living room and play the piano. There wasn't much else to do. There were books which we could read but we'd just sit and talk. That's the most we did!

"I was determined to get through the exams, which meant I had to study so I didn't go out in the nighttime. I had no interest in men because I was only interested in getting through. I got my orders when I went in training that I was to live the same life as I lived at home. My family was Methodist and we weren't allowed to dance. I could go to parties but not to dances, and dancing was healthy exercise, but they didn't see it that way and I wouldn't say to my parents, 'You don't know what you're talking about!' You didn't talk back! That was the way it was and I wouldn't disappoint my parents for the world. They were good parents but I missed out on a lot of fun. Other girls went out a lot and I don't know how they managed it. We were in a four-bed room and they'd come in and say, 'Tell us what you learned tonight, Grandy.' I'd say, 'I'm not telling you because while you were out having a good time, I was studying hard.' But then they'd say, 'When you tell us, we understand it better. You explain it better than the book.' And I was foolish enough to do it. But I never failed a subject, thank goodness!

"We got eight dollars after our probationary period. A big sum! But you know, we could buy stamps and writing paper and stuff like that. It didn't go very far but we were glad to even have that because people at that time didn't have a lot of money.

"After graduating I went home to Garnish to visit my family because I needed a vacation and I hadn't been home during training. To get to Garnish I went by carriage to Burin to connect with the boat. The boat couldn't get into the wharf in Garnish so they'd anchor and small boats would come out and get us and any supplies. I liked the boat but I was a poor sailor. My family couldn't do enough for me, they were so proud. My sisters were all married and there was only my brother and I who were single and I was there for his wedding. We loved him so much because he was the only boy. The Grand Bank Hospital had promised me that they would take me back as charge nurse when I finished, so while I was home, I went to see them. The doctor said, 'We have someone in your place.' I said, 'You promised me that if I went into training, I would have my position here.' He said, 'Well, we can't ask her to go,' and I said, 'I wouldn't expect you to,' because I knew that two nurses were too many. I said, 'Don't worry! I'm going back to St. John's where I'm sure of a position.' So I went back to Garnish, spent a couple of weeks with the family, and then packed my things and went to St. John's.

"I didn't have a job and was going to get an apartment, but I went to Cook Street which was a home for unwed mothers. I told them I was looking for a job and the nurse said, 'We can take care of you if you want to come here and work.' So I stayed because I got a room as the nurse there but I only stayed a month. I went to visit someone in the x-ray department at the Sanatorium and she asked me to take an x-ray because she didn't know too much about them. I did an x-ray course after graduation but didn't plan to spend my life doing x-rays and had only learned the bare necessities. I helped her do the x-ray on the patient and Dr. Peters came in. He said, 'You're not working here.' I said, 'No, sir, I was asked to help with this x-ray.' He asked if I knew x-rays and I told him I did the course. He said, 'Would you like a job? We can take you on here. We have an x-ray traveling clinic.' They had several nurses but nobody who could x-ray. I agreed to do it because it filled in the time and I needed the money. Setting up the equipment was always a big problem. We usually set up in classrooms but one community didn't have a place big enough so we x-rayed outdoors which was much better with lots of fresh air.

"I didn't know I was going to have to drive the van, but the people who owned garages taught driving and you got your license if you could drive around. I drove that van for years! Fixing flat tires was part of my driving course. If we got a flat tire, I fixed it. I'd put on the spare and stop at a garage, but there were so few garages that if we got another flat, we were out in the cold because we had no way to fix it. The tires had an inner tube and we managed with our wrenches and pump.

"We had good times. We stayed in boarding houses when we were traveling, which were the best places because the department picked them out. The people fed us royally because they respected nurses and nothing was too good for us so we were on our best behaviour! We did x-rays until five or six o'clock and went back to our boarding house. Our area was the Avalon Peninsula, which was quite enough because the roads weren't paved and the dust! We wore navy blue uniforms and by the time we got home, they were grey uniforms. It was interesting and I enjoyed it.

"We came back to St. John's on Saturdays where we had rooms on Water Street west. Saturday wasn't a day off because we had to develop x-rays in the dark room in the van. We took care of everything on Saturday and Sunday and were out on the road again on Monday. I always said I'd never work for the government and I worked with them all my lifetime.

"Eventually the Tuberculosis Association took over the mobile clinic so we didn't go out anymore. They visited places by boat that you couldn't get to by car. I would love to have gone but I got seasick so I wouldn't be much help! I worked with the mobile x-ray clinic from 1938 to 1940 and after that stopped, I did district nursing.

"In 1950, Dr. Peters was going to the new West Coast Sanatorium in Corner Brook and asked me to come with him and I worked there until 1963. I did x-rays the first year I was there. The Director of Nurses was from Vancouver but she was a bit bossy and Dr. Peters wasn't having any of that. It didn't bother me because she wasn't in charge of x-ray, I was. Dr. Peters called me in one day and said, 'I've got a new job for you. You're going to be the Director of Nurses.' I said, 'I couldn't do that and besides I have a good job.' He said, 'Oh yes, you can, and you're going to do it. After all, I'm the boss.' But it worked out and the nurses were wonderful to me.

"I didn't know a lot about the hospital but I thought about what I would like so I had them visit my office every week and we went over the work. It was necessary to get to know the staff. I'd visit the units and they never knew when I was coming. When they'd hear me walking up the stairs, I'd hear the young ones say, 'She's coming!' Then they'd all be busy at their work and no one sitting down except those doing the charts. I thought, 'I must be putting fear into them.' I was strict but I got on well with the nurses. They were a grand bunch and certainly gave good nursing care. It was a big responsibility because I was on call all the time. I had the phone by my bedside in case something happened, but the nurses spared me and wouldn't call unless it was absolutely necessary.

"My life became lonelier then because it's lonely being at the head. I would have liked to be working with another nurse but Dr. Peters gave me a lot of support. His wife Ruth was a great friend but she worked in the lab so she wasn't under my control.

I would have preferred to make friends with the nurses, but the hospital expected me to stay apart from the staff because if I was too friendly, they wouldn't do their work properly. They might think, 'We know her and we'll get off with that!' I think it was necessary but it was a lonely life and I couldn't let them off with things.

"I belonged to whatever groups I could and went to church functions. I made a lot of friends there and we had lots of fun and laughs. Even there, I couldn't get off with anything because they put me in charge of that too! I must say they did show me respect. I had my own apartment up on the hill with a little garden patch and I liked being able to plant things. Other staff, like the housekeeper, who lived in the residence, also planted and we'd see who could get the best patch. Because I wasn't in charge of them, I could be natural with them.

"When we opened the Sanatorium, we began to admit patients. Some of them were desperately ill and not able to move around, but others were a bit too lively and we had to keep an eye on them. If not, they were out running around. We had rest periods twice a day, one hour in the morning and one hour in the afternoon, and there was no talking. If they couldn't sleep, they had to lie quietly but few complained. They weren't supposed to do anything because even reading something exciting could cause their heart to beat faster. Some would sneak out to the bathroom and others could be destructive, like beating up the bathroom, so the nurse had to make rounds. We had two and four bedrooms and singles for the very sick, and all the doors had windows so we could see into the rooms. We knew it was hard on patients but those were the rules. They had to rest!

"The treatment for TB then was rest and drugs. A lot of patients liked going out on the veranda, so I asked Dr. Peters if the nurses could move their beds out during rest period on sunny days.

He thought it was a good idea, so we wheeled the beds out each morning and lined them up. The patients loved being outside but if anybody didn't want to go out, no one forced them. The patients could see all over Corner Brook from the veranda. They could even see people playing golf on the golf course. We'd put the head of their bed up a little bit and that satisfied them. We gave them something to drink so it was like a picnic. They'd have their dinner outside and we'd let them stay out after rest period.

"We'd only put out the children we could depend on, and we practically had one nurse to a child because we were very careful with little ones. When the little ones didn't have much, the staff would use their free time to buy things for them and then they would do them up, especially the girls, which was wonderful. They only saw their parents during visiting hours but they got a lot of love from the staff.

"The patients' food was fairly good. They had a dietician and we ate the same food as the patients. They would bring mine over to my apartment there because the lady in charge would always say, 'You're tired, I'll bring your meal over to you.' I preferred it that way, because you couldn't become familiar with people. How could I go in the dining room and not talk to them? You had to sort of stand off. You couldn't help it. It wasn't that I wished to be that way. I was expected to be dignified.

"Some patients didn't see their families for a long time because very few could afford to travel. You had to be 16 years old to visit because we couldn't afford to have TB spread, and the first thing a child would do is to go over and kiss Mommy. The parents only saw their children if they were sent pictures and very few had cameras in those days. So many of the women cried and we tried to help, but what can you do for people who are missing their children and their husbands? It was heartbreaking! We told the patients they could always talk to us and we kept them informed. Most of them could write and we provided stationery and stamps. The church played an important role and we'd ask the clergy to come in and talk to them. Some of the patients felt better if they could see their priest. Certain groups would go to Sunday mass and others had services with their clergy which they enjoyed and wouldn't miss. But we couldn't control the separation!

"We had a group that catered to the patients and taught them skills so some of them enjoyed being there. They did learn a lot and did sewing and knitting. It used to get me down. But they had clubs for them. The Rotary was grand at that. They'd have singing and they'd have games. They used to play a lot of Scrabble. They'd have concerts for the patients and the ones that were well enough would be allowed to come down and the others could hear it over the PA system.

"Dr. Peters' home was near and I visited them because I could talk to Ruth. She was a lovely person. I never could have done it if they hadn't been there to back me up. He was good to the patients and we all respected him. I worked at the Sanatorium from 1950 to 1963, thirteen years and I loved it. I left there and started housekeeping in North Sydney with my sister because we had sold our home in Garnish and my other sister had also gone to North Sydney.

"It's difficult to say if I'd do it again but I enjoyed doing it at the time. The training was very, very strict but you never neglected a patient. I loved nursing and I loved caring for people, especially the very ill. I wasn't an angel, by any means, but I enjoyed nursing."

CHAPTER 11:

Marjorie Hudson

"A nurse can make or break a hospital."

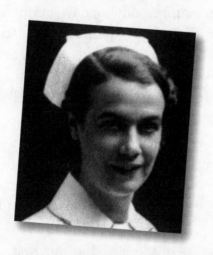

Marjorie Hudson [Moores Janes] graduated from the Grace School of Nursing in 1936 and worked there for most of her nursing career. Aside from a few years in administration, Marjorie preferred bedside nursing and the contact with her patients.

Majorie Hudson was one of five children. Her family had a little store in St. John's, which she says "kept them going."

"After I finished first-year intermediate, Mr. King, the

principal of Stanley Hall, wanted me to do grade 11 without doing second year intermediate because he thought I was wasting my time. I told him I wanted to stay with my friends who were going to do commercial. I tried commercial, but didn't like it. I was working with a chartered accountant when we had the tidal wave. The pictures began to move and I didn't know what was happening because it was over so quickly.

"You could get into nursing with grade 10, but my sister was in England on holiday from India and she came home here and told me to get my grade 11. She said, 'You won't regret it.' Mr. King made arrangements for me to do English and history matriculation exams in night school and physics in summer school. That was grinding, studying day and night! I had six labs a week, with one on Saturday. My mother or dad would bring up my lunch and we'd have birch beer and cookies. Sometimes a crowd of us would go to our house to get lunch. When I got my grade 11, I wore my school uniform as proud as could be!

"My sister was the first lady doctor in Newfoundland. She graduated from Edinburgh in 1937 and went to India as a medical missionary. I didn't consider medicine because I knew we couldn't afford it and I had two brothers coming up. I always wanted to be a nurse, so I went into nursing and loved it. I had an excellent training!

"We did dietetics at Memorial in our first year and we were supposed to be there at 7 p.m. but they would not let us off until quarter to seven and we'd run across LeMarchant Road like a blue streak because there were no taxis and we had no money. Doctors taught all our classes except practical nursing, which was taught by Ethel Barter. We stood whenever we met a doctor. If we were sitting at the desk or in the classroom, we stood because we respected them. We had Dr. Wilkinson and Dr. Blackler. Dr. Blackler never gave a mark if we left out 'ands' or 'buts' and he failed three out of eleven in my class. If a second-year student failed a subject, she had to repeat first year, but if you failed a subject in third year, you only had to repeat that subject. We had good lectures in the caseroom. Dr. Will Roberts trained us the way he thought we should be trained but he made us cry. He used to hammer Kate and I! Once we had a string of safety-pins for the T-binders and Kate and I strung them on a belt for a laugh. Dr. Roberts went to Miss Barter and said, 'Separate those two!' He gave me 52% in my skin diseases examination, but they had put me on nights because someone was sick and I wrote the exam in the next morning. I had been going to cram that night, but I was too sleepy. I often felt I got a raw deal because they'd send me here or there if someone was sick. They wouldn't care that I had been on all day or had to go on that night. They were good to us but we had to toe the line! We wouldn't think about quitting. We often said we'd quit, but you wouldn't think of doing it!

"In first year, we got off from ten to twelve but temperatures were taken at 10 a.m., and they had to be finished before you left! You never questioned the rules! One day, Miss Benson told me to take a man's temperature, but I was busy, so I said I couldn't do it. She said, 'You get busy and go right in.' My face was so red! Sometimes we cried because we thought we were right but they said we were wrong. Discipline was very important! Miss Benson would sit at the desk and if we passed she always gave us something to do. You could be getting a drink for the patient and you'd meet Miss Benson and she'd give you a different job immediately. If you had the glass in your hand, you'd put it down and do what she asked. You couldn't say, 'Well I got to go back.' We never talked back, even if we were right.

"We got up at six; prayers at six–thirty; and on the floor at seven. We worked seven to seven, seven days a week, and got off one Sunday from 10:30 a.m. to 2:30 p.m. and 2:30 to 6:30 p.m. on the next Sunday. Sometimes we got two hours off in the morning, but if we had a class, we only got one hour off and we only had one late leave a week. We never got off on time because we had to finish our work before we got off. If you had a half day you didn't have enough time to go home. Miss Ethel Barter would put us on nights and we wouldn't know we had to work that night until twelve o'clock. You came off nights in the morning, which was your day off, and went back to work the next day. I did six to eight weeks on nights without a break and they forgot I was on. You'd get off at four-thirty on Christmas Eve and wouldn't get home until five-thirty. You'd have to eat your Christmas dinner then get ready to go back to work. We had boyfriends, although we didn't see them very often and some of them were at university so they had to study. Sometimes we went to movies, and church was very important.

"We lived in residence and we had to be in ten o'clock on weeknights, ten-thirty Sunday nights, and one night at twelve o'clock. The butter company was next to the hospital and on the front there was a great big cow which was lit up and the light went out at ten. Jake Reid was the orderly who tended the furnace and other things. One night Dunne came in at ten o'clock, she thought, but the door was locked. She said to Jake, 'You locked the door before ten o'clock,' and he said, 'No, I didn't. The cow didn't have a late leave tonight!'

"I lived in St. John's, about a five-minute walk from the Grace, but I had to get out of uniform before going home on my time off. We weren't allowed out with our uniform on or we would be penalized. We wore our cuffs to meals and prayers, but we didn't wear them when we were doing work, and someone was always there to steal them. We got no money in the first six months and eight dollars a month for the three years. We'd go down to the Chinese laundry on Pleasant Street to get our belts, caps, and cuffs starched.

"Miss Benson was always five minutes early and one morning when she was having prayers, the bell rang and it wasn't quite half-past six. We got there just as prayers started but we were marked late and lost our free time. We all got together and decided we were going to be on time the next morning because Miss Benson was having prayers again. We went to bed and I woke up in the middle of the night thinking it was six o'clock, and I heard Miss Benson talking to Evelyn Roberts in the next bedroom. I woke up the girls in my room and we woke up the girls in the other room. We were making so much racket putting on our uniforms that Miss Benson came out and said, 'Where are you going?' We said, 'Going to prayers,' and she said, 'It's only one o'clock!'

"As students our day went quickly because we didn't have time to think. We started baths immediately and ran to the bathroom to get pans of water for the patients. We dry mopped the rooms, dusted, and made beds. We washed the transoms, which were the windows above the door. Everything had to be neat and tidy before breakfast. If we had an accident come in or a very sick patient, one of the nurses had to sit with the patient and then things were late. We couldn't go off until our charts, dressings, and patient care were done. One night two of us were on duty and an accident came in. One of the patients died and we didn't get off until ten o'clock the next morning because we had to do our charts and dressings before the day shift came on. Nobody complained, because everyone did it. It was expected! Nobody ever had to say, 'Help me,' because we just did!

"We had to do all the cleaning then, and I'd wear myself out carbolizing a bed because I used so much strength getting it clean. We learned to shroud patients and get them ready for burial. We'd bathe them just as if they were alive, pack their nose, ears and mouth. Then we'd dress them in their clothes, underwear and all. The caskets were brought to the hospital because only the undertakers buried them. I had one patient die and a student was helping me get her ready. We were talking in the hall, talking when the bell rang in the patient's room! We didn't say a word, just looked at each other and went in together. We were so scared! The bell had fallen off the bed!

"The hospital was small then, with only two floors, the case-room was on the first floor and the OR with the T and A room, we called it for tonsils and adenoids, on the other end of the hall. When we worked on the first floor, patients had castor oil every third morning and I hated it when we came on! Oh, the bedpans! Ethel Barter would say, 'Go, find Miss Hudson please, because she knows who is to have castor oil this morning.'

"The patients would have four and five pillows, one under their knees, their bottom, and two or three under their heads. It was a wonder we didn't kill them! We'd have two nurses lift a patient to avoid breaking any stitches. Then after lunch, we washed patients' face and hands and rubbed their backs and did it all again before we went off.

"Patients would come in with lice, and one time we had to cut a little girl's curls off. We had her mother's permission but she nearly had a fit! Another patient came to the OR with lice crawling on the pillow. The nurse who looked after her lost her cap because she didn't clean her hair.

"I was on surgery and coming off duty one day when Miss Thomas said, 'Rupert R. needs an enema.' He had a ruptured appendix and not many survived that in those days. There were no antibiotics and the treatment was a hot water bag on the abdomen for one hour then an ice bag for one hour. He developed peritonitis. Elsie Warren, who was senior nurse in the OR, told me they were going to do Rupert's surgery at two-thirty. I was going off at six-thirty but Miss Barter said, 'Come back at ten-thirty tonight to sit with Rupert.' He had a colostomy done and I had to record any vomit in the emesis dish. I looked into the dish and here were two long worms! I thought I was going to die!

We cleaned his colostomy with green liquid and kept changing him but the worms kept crawling out! I bet 20 came out of him, but he never got out of sorts even though no one gave him any hope. They gave up on him a dozen times but he survived. Doctor Jameson came in from a banquet one night with his tux on and said, 'I don't think I'll start that IV. It's no use.' But he put it in. Every afternoon when I'd wake up, I'd ask, 'Is Rupert alive?' Usually only senior students cared for really sick patients, but Crummy and I were on with him for four weeks even though we were only second years. His father and mother visited three times, but the third time they said they couldn't afford to come anymore. We told them we would write them every week. When Rupert went up to get his colostomy sewn up, Dr. Will Roberts said, 'Is there anything you'd like before the operation?' Rupert said, 'I'd like a chew-blow,' and Dr. Roberts sent one of the nurses to the store to get bubblegum, but Rupert never got spoiled. The day he left the hospital we were all in the main entrance. We were so proud of ourselves. I was working in the CSR in the 1950s when somebody came in and said, 'There's a man out here looking for a Nurse Hudson, who worked here years ago.' I went out and this was Rupert in to have a hernia repaired.

"When I worked on the children's ward, Dr. Will Roberts always told us to read the patients' histories when they were admitted. There were 42 children on the ward and he'd take the charts during rounds and asked me if the patient vomited, or if bowels moved, and things like that. He'd always check the time slip and if Ethel Barter was off, he'd come back in the afternoon to make rounds. He came in one day and everyone was gone except me. I was frightened to death but I had read their histories. Later, when I was in Outpatients, the nurses would come down to refill the drugs and they wouldn't know what was wrong with their patients. I'd say, 'Take the chart and read their history.' Oh, I had learned!

"We had a little fellow on the children's ward named Arthur who was a diabetic with a big stomach. He'd say to me, 'Huddy, will you give me my needley, please?' He'd go home and be back in no time in a diabetic coma. One night Gushue, the night supervisor, told me he was in and I went to see him. The first thing he said was, 'Huddy, will you give me my needley?' But Gushue said, 'No, she can't give you your needley.' He cried and went into a diabetic coma but I don't know if that was the cause. I was the first one he saw when he came out of it and he said, 'I love you, Huddy.' The youngsters got so attached to us that they cried when they had to go home.

"We sat with patients who had pneumonia, and children with pneumonia were put on the veranda with stocking caps, scarves, gowns, and socks on. They got fresh air just like in the San. If they had to be changed, we brought them into the ward, changed them, then put them back out again. One night I was sitting with a woman who had pneumonia and I had on a long gown, my cape, gaiters, and cap. The window was open and the wind would blow you out on the street! It was enough to freeze you! On the ninth day, we weren't allowed to take our eyes off the patient's face because that was the critical day. Either they recovered or not. Patients with pneumonia were treated with MB693s, which came in during my last year. We also used mustard plasters and linseed poultices and had to make those.

"A few years ago, I met a woman who asked me, 'Was your name Moores?' I said, 'Yes.' She said, 'Twenty-eight years ago, you dressed my little girl in Outpatients for six months.' Her daughter had spilled boiling water over her back and came to the Outpatients Department after discharge to get her skin graphs dressed. If I was off when the child came in, she'd go home because I'd always say to her, 'You can cry a little bit because it's going to hurt. We don't mind if you shed a few tears.' She'd say the same to her dolly. And I'd give her the adhesive and gauze ends to play with.

"We'd laugh and cry every day and we were sent to the office so many times for every little thing. I put the caseroom sheet up the wrong way and had to go to Major Fagner's office. She gave me a good lecture and told me I wasn't watching what I was doing. I shed a few tears but shedding tears was nothing. One night I was on the children's ward with 42 patients and by the time I got all the temperatures taken, it was time to go off duty. They wanted me to stay on with an isolation patient even though I wasn't a senior nurse but I said I was going home. They called my mother and she had to come up!

"We used to carry vials of morphine tablets in our pockets. We used a Bunsen burner to melt the morphine and had to record who we gave it to. Usually we gave 6 minims of tincture of digitalis so many times a day. Dr. Browning always wanted a milk and molasses enema for his patient before surgery, and we hated this because it wasn't supposed to curdle, but it did more times than not. There was a good stock of emergency supplies on all floors but we could also get drugs in a hurry from LeMarchant Drugs.

"We had three gas burners and had to boil the instruments on one of those. Dinner trays came up at eleven-fifteen and Major Fagner said, 'Whatever is on the gas jet at eleven-fifteen, comes off and the kettles go on. One day I had to put the kettles on and Sadie Ash was boiling instruments for some doctor. I took them off and was she angry! I never took things off again.

"Cass and I were in the same room in residence and one night Miss Thomas sent up for us. I wasn't working on the first floor so I didn't go. Cass came back and said, 'Miss Thomas said to get up.' So I got up and went over and they gave us a caseroom bundle and off we went in a taxi. This was two or three o'clock in the morning and we didn't know where we were going! We ended up in a house on Waldegrave Street where they only had a bed, an orange crate, and a stove with a pan of water on it. The patient never did deliver her baby and we were worn out looking at her. We phoned Miss

Thomas who got in touch with Dr. Carnell. We came back to the hospital at six-thirty, put on our uniforms, went down to breakfast and then went on duty.

"In maternity, we had to have seventeen deliveries without a doctor. If your patient got a perineal tear the doctor would have to suture it, and he'd look at you pretty badly so you put hot compresses on right away. One of the doctors told Stella, 'That woman won't deliver for another two to three hours, so I'm going off now.' Stella got un-scrubbed and went to dinner. The next thing I knew the baby came! I had gloves on, but forgot to take off my watch! I rang the caseroom bell to get somebody from the floor. When she came back, all Stella could think about was that I wasn't scrubbed. The two of us cried that day!

"Dr. Nigel Rusted kept his maternity patient in the hospital two or three days longer than other doctors, and he didn't let them get up for nine days after delivery. He did the same for his surgical patients. Hernia patients were fed for twenty-one days so we hated to see a hernia patient come in! Dr. McPherson always walked his patient from the caseroom to her room. We thought he was crazy but he was right! ─────────

"We were very professional on duty and the only time I wasn't was when Dr. Rusted had a patient with two burned breasts. He ordered dressings every four hours which took about two hours to do. I said to Dr. Rusted, 'I only get the dressings on when we have to take them off again.' He hadn't realized that so he changed the order to every eight hours. The woman wasn't getting any benefit because we were disturbing the tissue changing the dressings so often.

"We affiliated at the Fever. We'd get patients with typhoid, diphtheria, scarlet fever, and measles. There were pans of water everywhere because we had to wash our hands. We washed them a thousand times a day! The Fever was an old building and they had cats around because of mice. One day, a cat jumped up on me and frightened the wits out of me!

"I was in my last year when King George VI died. We were in the lecture room studying for an exam, and they came and told us. The next day we had to wear black and purple ribbon on our sleeves.

"I graduated in 1936, but they only had a graduation every second year because they couldn't afford it, so our ceremony was for 1936 and '37. We didn't mind because there was only eleven in our class and we had a nice graduation.

"After graduation, they wanted me to go in charge on surgery, with Ethel Barter as assistant supervisor, but it was a lot of responsibility and I didn't want it so I did private duty. I went back part-time on staff some time later, but I was up in administration for two or three years and I didn't much care for it because I didn't have any patient contact. I wanted to be in contact with the patients, so I'd make rounds. One day I went on one of the floors and an old lady couldn't reach her tray because they didn't lower her table! Another day I went to the third floor and an old lady with pneumonia was sitting in the chair with her chin on her chest and the nursing assistant was making the bed! I said, 'Should she be up this hour in the morning without her breakfast?' She said, 'I don't know.' So I said, 'I'll help you make the bed and we'll get the patient back in it as quickly as possible.' I went out to the Head Nurse and said, 'I thought the grads looked after the really sick patients because I just went into a private room and the nursing assistant has a very sick patient up in the chair and she can't keep her head up. If she were my mother, she'd be out of here in five minutes! Where are the grads?' She said, 'They're talking to the patients in the bathroom.' I met the Head Nurse the next day and she told me that the woman was the mother of one of the doctors and she had told him what I said!

"The patients gave us little presents in appreciation. Private patients paid four dollars a day, and if they were in a private ward with a bath between they'd pay five dollars a day. Carrie Jameson and I did private duty with Reverend Baggs who was critically ill. He got many tablets every half hour and Carrie would come in at six o'clock in the morning and shout at him to wake him. He'd jump a mile! When I was on duty he'd say, 'When you give me pills, you rub my hand to wake me up but she yells!'

"Cummings and I were on with a German captain who died just before Cummings came on duty at eight o'clock. I told her he had died and while we were talking, he made a big burp. I tell you, we were frightened out of our wits! But it was just the air coming out of his lungs.

"My father put the first radio sets in the Grace Hospital, and the patients used the headphones to hear services and the radio. One night Don Jameson was at the hospital and met a crowd of women standing by a patient's door. He asked them what they were doing and they said, 'We're waiting to see how we are tonight!' Every night on the Gerald S. Doyle news, it was announced how patients were doing in the hospital, what they had done that day or were going to have done.

"I'd go back to nursing. I enjoyed it all. We had our ups and downs; that was normal but we didn't mind hard work. It was better than sitting around wondering what to do. We were poorly paid, but we didn't mind that either. Nurses are not paid enough for what they have to go through."

CHAPTER 12:

Eileen Shanahan

"I really had no problem [in nursing] but mind you, I said my prayers, more often than not, that everything would turn out all right… When you're on your own it's kinda scary, you know."

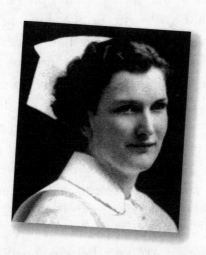

Eileen Shanahan [Thorburn] was born in Harbour Grace in 1912 and graduated in 1937 from the 18-month Midwifery Program at the Grace Maternity Hospital. After graduation she completed a public health course and additional midwifery training while doing district nursing in St. John's. She was the Nurse-in-Charge of the Old Perlican Cottage Hospital when they began to do surgery there and introduced sterile technique to the OR. She also worked as District Nurse in Grand Brit before she married and raised nine children.

Eileen Shanahan was one of nine children. It was her involvement in the care of her siblings that she credits for her decision to go in nursing. "From about three years of age, I was really interested in caring, looking after the children in my mother's family. When I was ten or eleven I read everything about nursing to find out all about it. Then my young brother had his appendix out at the Grace and my mother stayed with him. She was so delighted with the care that she came home and said, 'Put in your application.' I applied to the Grace and I was also trying to get sent to Peter Brigham Hospital in Boston, but my father said I couldn't go there but I could go to the Grace. During the Depression, we didn't have much money but we had to have money for our uniforms and we managed. As students we got pin money, which was eight dollars a month and you'd be surprised what we got out of that. I'm delighted I went to the Grace. The discipline was better there than anywhere. I was thrilled and treated extremely well by Miss Fagner and Miss Barter, the whole staff. I think I was the first one from my community that went to be a nurse, and I was finished and had three or four children before the next one from the same area went in training. I was 21 when I went in nursing because I did a business course first. When we'd go to our nursing classes they'd say, 'You do them in shorthand.' Then they'd copy my notes.

"It was unusual for Catholic students to go to the Grace hospital but St. Clare's wasn't a training school then. There were five of us in our group. At six o'clock, we'd go to assembly for prayers and a hymn to start the day but they excused us. But that didn't affect our training or our respect and love for the Grace. We were just one happy family and delighted to be there. There was a Gabriel Hannon who trained with me, and Miss Fagner never called me anything but Miss Hanashan. It was so funny. She knew there was another person with a name something like mine but she always got the two of us mixed up. I got four hours off on Sunday and Miss Fagner would say, 'Now, Miss Hanashan, you have to go to your church this morning.' I'd go for ten o'clock and be back at eleven, then go back on duty at three. I had no complaints. I'm still very proud of the Grace.

"I was a probationer, only in about a month, and I was called back on duty because someone got sick and had to go off. There was a patient who was coughing and coughing and Miss Fagner's office was on the same floor. She came out of her office and said, 'Will you give that patient two grams of *creoterpen*?' We did the metric system in pharmacology and had to know it for our exam. I poured an ounce and brought it into the patient. That's an honest fact! She said, 'That's a lot to take,' and I said, 'You have to take every drop.' I was going to get her another ounce but she said, 'Nurse, that's plenty. I'll go to sleep now.' I was frightened to death to tell anyone because I didn't know what *creoterpen* was. I told the nurse on the floor and she said, 'That's fine, it won't hurt her. I don't think it'll make any difference.' But I was worried to death and didn't sleep the next night. I said, 'Do I have to tell Miss Fagner?' But she said, 'Write down one ounce and if it's questioned, you can answer it.' I think Dr. Will Roberts made reference to it, but Miss Fagner didn't know; it didn't get to her. The patient went home to Bell Island and wrote me to find out what medicine I gave her because she hadn't coughed since. The amusing part was that she wanted to get more of the medication. She couldn't get it on Bell Island so she wanted me to send it, which I didn't. I wrote her and said, 'Go to the pharmacist in Bell Island. He'll give you something and follow the directions.' That was the only mistake I ever made.

"We did twelve hours, seven to seven, and were taught that you didn't go and leave any unfinished work for the nurse coming on. I distinctly remember one day on obstetrics we were really busy. I said to Miss Thomas, 'I'm not going to take my two hours free time. The caseroom has to be cleaned and a lot of things are left to be done.' She said, 'I'm so thankful.' But the next day she made me take my two hours: 'You take what you deserve.' I loved her; she was a darling. I liked Miss Benson a lot too. She was a very clever lady with a big responsibility. I was kind of nervous about Miss Benson so I used to avoid passing her. You'd have things to do like clean the bathrooms, get surgical trays ready for the doctors or dressings, and if you passed her on your way to get something she'd have something else for you to do. You wouldn't dare say, 'I can't, Miss Benson, I have this to do.' You'd go and do it and finish the other thing later! That's the way it was and we never questioned it. When I worked in Kelowna the staff would always get upset with me because if things weren't finished, like orders not written or taken care of and everything not ready for the evening shift, I'd always stay. They'd say, 'Let the girls coming on do it,' but I couldn't do that. I'd say, 'That's the way I was trained and that's what I'm going to do.'

"We had boyfriends but we weren't allowed to go out with patients and you couldn't take money. I had a special private patient and he wanted to give me five dollars. I said to him, 'I'm sorry but I can't take it.' He went down to Miss Fagner and left the five dollars with her. She came up and gave it to me. He also asked me out for dinner at the Sterling Restaurant, which was the most popular one in St. John's. I said, 'I can't fraternize with patients.' He said, 'That's fine. I'll ask her if you can come.' I was getting off at seven o'clock and Miss Fagner told me, 'The gentleman you nursed wants to take you out to the dinner,' and he took me out. I had to be in by ten but we were late getting back because we went to see a show and it was late starting. That was one time I lost my late leave. Sometimes you would go for a drive after a show or go to the café across from the hospital, which closed at half past ten. Other than that we did very little socializing. One night three or four from our class went to a show; Ginger Rogers and Fred Astaire was playing. We'd warn the janitor if we were going to sneak in. This night he had the basement door open. When you went out in those days you wore a hat and gloves and you'd have to pull them off before you sneaked in bed. Miss Fagner would come down to check that we were in bed. This night we heard her coming and we jumped in bed with our clothes on and put the bed clothes up. Chris Dunn got in bed with her hat on and Miss Fagner just said, 'Miss Dunn, would you take off your hat?' We were seniors then. We had our escapades, got away with some but not with others. Sometimes we'd lose our late leaves. I lost mine a couple of times.

"I went in nursing in 1934 and finished 1937. When we finished training I got five dollars a week, so I was making a whole lot of money, going from eight to twenty dollars a month. There were no jobs but I was really very lucky. Miss Barter was in charge and she asked me to go in charge of the infant nursery. I was there for two months when I thought I'd apply to public health. I applied and did a year in the district. Although we got a wonderful obstetrical training at the Grace, I did midwifery while I was there. Miss Whiteside gave us the course in midwifery. You had a little funnel for doing the baby's heartbeat. You knew about the mother by the prenatal examination. You knew if there was anything wrong, such as the baby being in the wrong position, and you'd call the doctor right away. I think the doctor came once and put in a couple of stitches, but the way Miss Whiteside trained us, we thought it was mismanagement if we had a tear. We were mortified if one of our patients had a tear and I never had any in my practice. We'd have hot compresses ready and we thought they were the best method of all. You kept the hot compresses on until you'd see the head presenting and then you'd know they were ready to deliver. Of course we could always call the doctor if we ran into difficulty but we rarely did.

"We stayed at the Balsom Hotel when we took our course in public health and Miss Whiteside stayed there with us. She was very strict so we had to be on our p's and q's. Her meals were brought to her room. She didn't mix with us but she had friends on the S.S. *Newfoundland*, which came to St. John's from England, and she'd eat in the dining room with the captain and her friends when they came. Apart from that she had a pretty lonely life. I found Miss Whiteside to be a very special person. Mind you, when the doctors were there, they'd say, 'Don't mind her, she's English.' But she really knew what she was teaching us. She used to write me about once a month when I was in Grand Brit but then she went back to England. When I worked in Kelowna, I had a patient who told me she had done a midwifery course in England from a Miss Whiteside. She was telling me how strict she was and how fearful they were of doing the wrong thing. I said, 'Hold it a minute, she taught us in Newfoundland!' I couldn't believe it! It really is a small world, isn't it?

"After my public health course I got $90 a month and had to pay 40 for board at the Balsom. I had the handsome sum of $50 left. I was really well off! While doing public health in St. John's, we'd be on call. They'd call the hotel if there was a delivery and two of us would usually go so there was an extra nurse to assist with the delivery, but if there weren't two available only one nurse would go. I was called to Signal Hill to do a delivery and the baby had spina bifida. Luckily I realised there was something wrong. At first it looked like I should have ruptured the membranes, but I thought, 'No, I'll let it go.' The woman was a Catholic and I just had time to baptize the baby when it died. Dr. Miller was in charge of Public Health and Welfare then. When I sent him my report, he sent for me and said, 'You take two days off and go where you want.' I suppose he thought it was a bit of stress and anxiety for me. That was the only bad experience I had while out in the district. Other than that, the experience was just fantastic, really marvellous. I was also nursing in the district during the war, going by myself after midnight. I was scared to death of anyone walking behind me. I often wonder now how I did it.

"During this time I gained confidence to go out and take over a district. I was sent to the cottage hospital in Old Perlican. I didn't go in charge right away but did later. In addition to the midwifery, I had also done dentistry from Dr. Royal because I was going to have to pull teeth while I was out there. We used to do five to eight tonsillectomies a day and I'd assist. I got information on how to make up and use the sterile lap sets from the Grace Hospital. I wrote Grace Alexander there and she sent me everything. I made the gowns, and I tell you, the sleeves were down to here because I never sewed before. I made up the lap sets for obstetrics and tonsillectomies. We did the first appendectomy at the cottage hospital in Old Perlican, and I assisted Dr. Strat who came from Harbour Grace and was fresh out of training. When he came to start the surgery I got the gloves and put his hand in. He said, 'What's this?' I said, 'You be careful and don't contaminate the gloves.' He said, 'You only see that in movies or hear about it on the radio.' Everything was done according to what I had learned in the Grace Hospital operating room. I'd get it all ready and say, 'This is what you do. Don't contaminate anything.' I had a man come in with a cut on his face. I called the doctor who was on his way to town and said, 'Come in before you go. This man needs about three stitches.' He said, 'Do it yourself,' and I did it. It looked all right too and the man was really happy about it.

"Sometimes Dr. J. King would come down from Northern Bay. He took a course in eye, ear, nose and throat and did several cases of tonsils in Old Perlican and I assisted. He'd say, 'You tell me what to do,' and he listened. I sort of felt I was in control and got their respect. They didn't know the things that a nurse would know; they only knew their own profession. I feel I did a good job there and I'm not boasting. I was really satisfied. I feel I set the standard.

"Old Perlican Cottage Hospital was like a closely knit family; it was wonderful. There weren't a lot of things to do socially but we used to go out to Dr. LeGrow's place and his wife would make us a lovely dinner. Laura Elliot also worked there; she was a nurse from the General. We had two nurses and two nurses' aides, Norrie March and a Miss Hodder. They knew just about as much as we did by the time they left, they were really good. I was there for nearly two years.

"Then I was transferred in charge of the district in Grand Brit. There were always men around the wharves and when I got off the boat, they said, 'Where are you going? You're new here.' I said, 'I'm coming to look after the district.' They said, 'My dear, are you finished school?' I said, 'Oh yes, I'm a graduate nurse.' The nurse before me was from England and in her forties. She was more experienced than I was, but I got along very well and I had a fully equipped surgery.

"I had a husband bring his wife in and he said, 'Sister, my wife is having a terrible time with her teeth. She'd like to have them taken out and I hear you can do it.' They called me Sister then. I said, 'Okay,' and got my dental outfit ready. I put her on the table and looked in her mouth and I said, 'So, how many teeth?' I wasn't sure but I thought there were about 10 or 12. I got things ready and pulled 12 teeth or little stumps. The husband said, 'Thank you very much, Sister. I can't afford to go to Dr. Heath (the doctor in charge in Burgeo). I went down with her to have them taken out a couple of months ago, but Dr. Heath said she'd have to stay three weeks because they had to take out one tooth at a time because she has a very bad heart.' Well I tell you, it frightened the daylights out of me! I said, 'You don't have to go back. Stay here and I'll give her an ounce of brandy.'(They lived way up the coast). I got a cot and got her settled. I put him on the examining table and they slept there for the night. I put in a big fire in the hall stove and every two or three hours I'd do her blood pressure and check how she was doing. It was a big shock! I told Dr. Heath about it later. I had to cable him a couple times and he'd cable back saying 'Stand on your own two feet, you can do it.' That gave me little bit of encouragement.

"I was there about two months when a man came to see me and said, 'This is my wife, she's having her first baby. If anything happens to her you're finished,' and I wondered what he meant by that. About quarter to two one morning, I got the call: 'Come over, my wife is ready. She's having a lot of pain.' I got everything ready and they were downstairs waiting. Finally she had a baby girl, seven or eight pounds. She had a little spot on the back of her head and I thought, 'He's going to kill me for this but it's not my fault.' I told him, 'You have a little daughter and there's a little bump on her head due to the pressure.' 'Never mind, Sister,' he says, 'the top of the kitchen door is too low for her head so she always bumped it going in and out. That's what caused that.' I said, 'No, it didn't, but the baby is fine.' A couple of days after the delivery, he came over to my boarding house and asked for me. I thought, 'My God, what's happened now?' He wanted to know my full name. I said, 'Eileen Shanahan.' He said, 'You must have another name.' I said, 'Yes, Eileen Mary Magdalene Shanahan.' He said, 'That's fine, my daughter is going to be called Eileen Mary Magdalene.' Now Grand Brit was strictly a United Church community and I was Catholic. I was surprised when he said, 'She's going to have your name.' I thought it was an honour.

"I really had no problem but, mind you, I said my prayers more often than not that everything would turn out all right. Miss Whiteside taught us well. We knew that if there was any problem, it was mismanagement. I always had that in the back of my mind when I was in the district but I enjoyed every minute. In Old Perlican, I had the doctor right there, but Dr. Heath was in Burgeo, which is a day and a half on a boat, and we had no phones. When you're on your own it's kinda scary, you know.

"I'd go on the boat from Grand Brit up to LaPoile and almost up to Port aux Basque to visit patients and the schools. I was really into health, so if the schools weren't tidy and clean I told them about it. Some of the teachers were really upset at first because I'd look at the toilets and say they'd have to be cleaned for health reasons. After a little while they thanked me for helping them.

"When we graduated from the Grace, we received our diploma from Lady Walwyn, who was the lieutenant governor's wife. There were 12 or 14 of us. When I came up to get my diploma, she shook my hand and said, 'That's my name, Eileen.' When I went back to my class and told them what she had said, they said, 'She never said anything to us.' When I went to Grand Brit and needed things, I thought, 'This is the lady I have to write.' I got whatever I wanted for the surgery, like instruments and clothes for children.

"The area was very poor. I was the only one who had a radio and there was a program with a lot of singing and dancing. The people would line up outside to listen to it. I'd open the window so they could hear the music and dancing. That was one happy thing, particularly for the school kids. I couldn't invite them in because all I had was a small bed sitting room but I enjoyed every bit of it.

"We lived in the hospital at Old Perlican but in Grand Brit I was in a boarding house. I didn't eat with the family. She passed my meals in through a little lift. That was the custom of the nurse before me. I didn't know anything about district work so I went along with it. Anyway, I don't think they wanted me to eat with them. The nurse was a special person in the community; she was very respected. When the people were talking, they were very guarded and would never say anything to offend you and they'd never ask questions. They'd just talk about themselves. The boarding mistress would say, 'What would you like to eat?' And I'd probably say chicken or for breakfast, maybe poached or boiled eggs. You didn't have much choice, but they got a lot of sea birds and fish and we'd have fish and turrs that were dressed. I liked them and you could have seconds. The boarding mistress was very kind to me because I had a finicky appetite and she was concerned about that. She'd say, 'You have to eat, I'll have to give you more and I won't raise your board money.' It cost me twelve dollars a month for board and lodging, three dollars a week. Can you imagine!

"It was lonely and I don't know how I filled my time. Once in a while I'd go to Burgeo and stay with the doctor and his wife, and I was invited out in the community maybe three or four times in all while I was there. I used to go skating on the pond with the young son from the boarding house who was about my age. He'd ask me and I was delighted to go rather than be stuck in during the evenings and nights. Some of the associations would have a get-together in the hall. I'd go to them but you just sat around and talked. Other than that there wasn't much to do socially. I used to read and review my nursing books.

"When I'd go out on a call with my bag, the boarding mistress would come to the door and say, 'What's wrong with Mrs. Smith.' Instead of saying 'I can't discuss it with you,' I'd say, 'I really don't know. I've only seen her once or twice.' Then they'd say, 'She doesn't know what she's doing because when you ask her what's wrong, she doesn't know.' All the doors would be opened with people asking 'What's wrong? How is she? Is she going to live?'

One time I heard them say, 'Sister was reading her book today. I think so and so has the measles but she's going to find out.' I didn't say anything because everything was strictly confidential with me. That was one thing I had to contend with because I couldn't tell them, but that didn't seem to deter them from questioning me. The boarding mistress would look in through the little shutter used to pass in my meals if somebody phoned and asked for me, she'd say, 'She's reading her book to see what's wrong.' But that didn't stop them from trusting me and they were really great.

"Once every two months I'd go with the minister and his wife to different outports and visit patients who couldn't get to the surgery. There would always be somebody at the boat to meet me and I enjoyed doing that because I'd meet other people. In Grand Brit, I'd open the surgery in the morning at half past eight or nine, then I'd have my lunch hour and go back until four or five, but they'd come at all hours if they needed to. I dispensed drugs. I had a little scale, my drug book and the recipes, and I made up iron and sodium compounds. I'd give out Blaud's pills, which were for the appetite and if you were run down. I didn't use many controlled drugs like sleeping pills.

"I only signed a one-year contract for Grand Brit and when it was up Miss Syretha Squires, who was in charge of Public Health wrote me and said, 'Come back and go in charge of cottage hospital in Old Perlican again because you know every nook and cranny.' I thought it over and was going to go, but I got married instead in 1941. So I never did get back to Old Perlican.

"I enjoyed every minute of my nursing, but I got married and had nine children so I couldn't do very much nursing after that. I did work in Kelowna General for about ten years, and then I retired."

CHAPTER 13:

Mary Galway

*"At that time they were starving for nurses in New York.
The papers were full of ads… We knew it wouldn't be any problem
to get a job because they were screaming for nurses."*

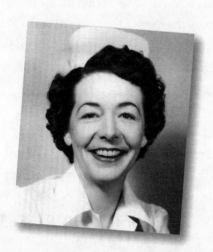

Mary Galway [Tucker] was born on August 31, 1915, in the capital of the country of Newfoundland to a close-knit family. She entered the General Hospital School of Nursing and found the experience overwhelming. She graduated in 1938. After brief working experiences at the Mental Hospital, Fort Pepperrell, Edmonton, and the General Hospital in St. John's, Mary moved to New York. Her great determination to improve nursing care, along with her outspoken manner, enabled her to demand higher standards. Her career accelerated from staff nurse to Head Nurse to Director of Nurses.

"I went to kindergarten at what is now St. Clare's Mercy Hospital; it was a private school at the time. After that I went to Mercy College and did primary and high school. I applied for nursing school before I graduated from high school but there were no vacancies. There wasn't a great deal of other things to do. That was during the Depression! I was one of ten children. I don't think we suffered but there were no jobs as such. People had very little money but my family really didn't suffer. We were quite comfortable. I always wanted to be a nurse and my family was very supportive. It took a long time, then eventually I did get in May '35 and finished in November '38. I finished school when I was 17, but I was nearly 20 when I entered nursing. I think most of the nurses were at least 19 because all the girls in my class were my age. There were only eight of us in our class.

"The first day I was terrified! Although I was one of ten children, I came from a sheltered home. Some of the language and some of the talk among the nurses when they were not on duty was coarse and I wasn't used to it. I didn't know these people. I had no friend there. I'd hear them out in the corridor, shouting and talking and I was in this room by myself. It was quite frightening, especially when you came from a large family where everybody was very close and very happy. It was a strange atmosphere but only the first little while.

"I really enjoyed the work but I thought, 'I don't know if I can stand this atmosphere.' One night I met my mother after duty. I knew all the work she had put in, all the uniforms she had made and all the aprons, but I said, 'Mom, I don't think I can stay down there any longer.' And she said, 'Well, if you can't, you come on home.' I think that was the best thing she ever said to me! I said, 'I'm going back and I'm going to stay!' After that I accommodated myself very well. There were long hours but I didn't mind the work. I used to hear the girls say they were tired and I really didn't know what that meant. The work didn't bother me as much as the complete change of environment and atmosphere.

"The uniform was a tight-fitting dress with long sleeves and no cuffs. It wasn't extremely long. We had separate bibs and aprons. We had an awful lot of aprons and bibs because you changed them every day. White shoes and stockings. The uniforms were done in the hospital laundry.

"The Matron was Miss Taylor and I remember her very well! She was a very, very strong, severe disciplinarian; that's all I can call her. There was no makeup or anything like that allowed on duty. I remember shopping one day and meeting her on Water Street and said, 'Hello, Miss Taylor.' The next morning I was called down to her office and she said, 'Did you have common [lipstick] on your lips when I met you yesterday?' Common! Red! I had to say 'Yes.' That will tell you how observant she was and how strict she was! I wasn't on duty. That didn't make any difference to her; I was called down to her office!

"We took anatomy, physiology, medicine and surgery and pediatrics. Dr. Bennett lectured us. Pat Gallagher and Dr. Kyle were interns there at the time. These were the people who gave us lectures as well as Dr. Murphy and Dr. Will Roberts. Nursing skills were taught on the floor. We went with a senior nurse, and she showed us how to make the beds and how to take care of the patients. Most of the floors had one graduate nurse, and the rest were students. There were senior students, intermediate students, and junior students. Our relationship was quite pleasant but you were supposed to stay at your own level. We had so little social life that it didn't really matter that much.

"We had to pack the linen at the back of the wards. Cowan and Crowdy, Shea and Carson, Victoria and Alexander – they were the main units in the hospital. Alexander was a children's ward, Victoria was the surgical floor. Cowan was women, and Crowdy, Shea, and Carson were male. The operating room was just a little area upstairs by the elevator. Now, there was an operating room off the Victoria Ward where they did tonsils or any dirty case that they didn't want to bring to the main operating room. I worked in the OR for two months during training. I didn't enjoy it much. To me the operating room was more of a mechanical thing than nursing. I worked more on the surgical floors where we had a lot of TB of the bone, hernias, appendectomies, hysterectomies, gastrectomies, and the usual surgical procedures.

"You were called at six o'clock, breakfast was at six-thirty and then you went to the floors about five minutes to seven and started to make beds. That was the routine – every bed was changed every day. The real sick patients got bed baths but not every patient got a bed bath every day by any means. Then breakfast was served and we had to bring in the trays. After breakfast, there were plenty of dressings to do especially for the patients with TB bone infections. Then there were patients to get ready for the operating room, giving enemas, and so on. By the time you'd take your break, the doctor would be ready to make rounds. There was always something to do – people coming back and forth from the operating room and you'd sit with them. While we were watching the patients recover from their anesthetic we'd make dressings to be sterilized, dry gloves, and powder them and get them ready for the autoclave. We'd send them to the operating room for autoclaving. There was no central supply when I was there.

"We had the usual painkillers. We had aspirin, morphine,

Demerol and Pentathol, and codeine, of course. At the time there were very few antibiotics. Sulfa drugs came in when I was in training. There was nothing like you have today, I can assure you.

"There were very few wound infections. A wound infection, in my day, was a horror – it was a disgrace! There were a lot of ruptured appendices and various things like that. I mean the dressings had to be changed. For the normal clean surgical procedure we didn't change the dressing, only when we took out the sutures – that was all. Patients were in bed until they had their sutures out, at least seven or eight days. A hernia was in bed for three weeks! When they got up, they were practically invalids! You can imagine the state of their muscles by the time they got out of bed. People were discharged and they could scarcely walk.

"I was Catholic so I never got a Sunday off because we had to go to mass at ten-thirty. We'd get off the ward at quarter to ten and then come back at one o'clock and work until nine o'clock. We were supposed to get a day off every two weeks but that didn't always happen because it depended on whether there was someone off for any reason. You didn't know until you came down in the morning and it would posted on the board if you had a day off. I'd sneak down about six o'clock to see if I could sleep in! But I never objected to any of that. It was no burden to me because once I got into the swing and adapted myself to the new environment, I was really quite happy.

"I think I was in training six months when I went on night duty. I was all alone with twenty-five to twenty-seven patients, depending on how many beds were down the center. Around five o'clock in the morning, you had to pass all these patients a basin of water and water to clean their teeth. We had a semi-private patient on the ward with a screen around his bed. There was an old gentleman who had leg amputation and was progressing very well. He was practically ready to go home. The day before had been his birthday and his family brought him down a cake. Before I started to distribute the pans of water, I went in to see him. I asked him if there was anything he wanted because I was going to be busy. He said he'd like a piece of cake. I went out and got a piece, propped him up in bed and put up his bedside table and passed him his cake. I went on about my business. After I was finished, I went in to look at him, and he was dead. Well, of course, immediately, I started to cry! I didn't know what else to do. I thought I killed him! I was devastated! There was another private patient across the room who was going to have surgery on his fractured elbow. He was going to be done that morning at eight o'clock, so when he found out the man was dead and I was crying and making a fuss, he said, 'Give me my pants, I'm getting the hell out of here!' He got his clothes and left for home. He went to his death with his straight elbow; he never had it done.

"There was a Salvation Army woman who came in to have a breast amputated in the morning. Back then we had to comb every head before the patient went to the operating room. This woman's hair was really in a bad shape. I said, 'What am I going to do with this woman's hair in order to get all the lice out?' Even though I was only a student I took the scissors and cut her hair. Her husband came in and he raised holy ructions because her hair was cut. Apparently, people in the Salvation Army weren't allowed to have their hair cut short. He went to Miss Taylor, and even though I was on night duty, I was awakened the next morning to go see her! I said to Miss Taylor, 'There was no other answer. I didn't know what I could do with the woman. She was going to the operating room the next morning and had extremely long hair and it was *lousy*! I had to cut it.' She must have pacified the man because it was the last I heard of it.

"One of the girls in our class was in the operating room. A child had his tonsils out and she picked up scabies from the child and we all picked it up from her and I even brought it home. All ten of the family got it and I was ready to be ostracized! A lot of the girls brought it home. Mary, another student, had two or three single aunts who lived with her mother and she brought it home to all of them. We all were ostracized!

"We really had very little social life. Someone would come down and pick you up outside the door because there was no telephone contact. You weren't allowed to take a telephone call on duty unless it was some kind of emergency. Don't forget, I had a couple of years of social life after I got out of school. They'd come down to wait for you, and they'd wait for you, and eventually, they'd have to *go* because you didn't show up. It was nothing to have to stay on the wards until eight o'clock.

"Miss Taylor was the Director of Nursing. We saw her every day when she made rounds but she died while I was in training. I think she died from a ruptured appendix or something simple like that. I'd say she died in '38. Because of that we never did have a graduating ceremony. We just finished. Then Mabel Smith took over as the Director of Nurses. She was Head Nurse on one of the floors and was a very capable woman. She was a great girl to get organized and get things done.

"My last affiliation was at the Mental. They were about to start insulin therapy as shock treatment. Dr. Reid asked me to work on that floor when I finished. I was pretty good at giving intravenous and so he asked me do that therapy. Kay Fraser from the General worked there. We worked together and I enjoyed it very much. I stayed there for about a year. They tried this treatment on all types of manic-depressives and schizophrenics. I think we gave insulin to about twelve patients at a time. We were down in the unit by ourselves and the patients were brought down each morning, and we gave them insulin in gradual doses until they went into convulsions. We'd let them have the first convulsion and then bring them out with glucose intravenous. It was kind of a drastic treatment. We didn't have good results with the schizophrenics but we had very good results with the manic-depressives. That's before they started electric shock.

"The male section was on the other side of the hospital and conditions there were appalling. The first floor had ambulatory patients and they were all in fairly good shape. Some of them probably shouldn't have been there, but in those days, most people abandoned their mentally ill people. Dr. Reid asked me to go over there and try to improve the conditions. The patients would sit at a large wooden table and they would bring in galvanized buckets of food. They would ladle the food out on tin plates. It was appalling! I got tables, tablecloths, and dishes and had them bring in vegetable dishes. I did a lot of that kind of thing to try to make it a little more humane. They loved it! You'd be surprised by the reaction. They felt that someone was doing something for them. Around '39 or '40, it was Commission Government. It was almost impossible to get anything out of the government or to make any changes. Dr. Reid was a very progressive man for his time. He investigated many of the patients' histories and that was never done before. He tried to find answers and tried to improve the conditions of mental patients."

The arrival of the Americans in Newfoundland opened up opportunities for nurses. Mary began to work at Fort Pepperrell. She describes the differences in working conditions: "Well… for one thing, we had shorter hours. You worked an eight-hour day and knew when you were getting your day off. There was no comparison in the salaries, although that was not important to me. At the General Hospital or the Mental Hospital, you made $53 a month. At the base, we made $150; quite a difference! When I went to work at Fort Pepperrell in 1941, they were getting the patients out of bed right after an operation. That was a surprise to me.

They were a little more advanced. The Director of Nurses was an American woman, but the staff nurses were practically all from the General Hospital or the Grace. I worked there in the surgical unit until February '43 when the unit closed. The doctors who worked there were transferred to Edmonton, Alberta, and asked three of us to go with them so I went.

"In Edmonton I worked in the Outpatient Department and really enjoyed it. There was only a small staff. I wasn't very fond of Western Canada. At the time, Edmonton was a very small country town; there was one main street, one hotel, and I had enough of it and I missed my family. I became engaged out there. He was a doctor in the army and was going back to be reassigned so I came home. I was in Edmonton from May to the following July.

"I was only home a very short time when they called me from the General Hospital to know if I would relieve for a month; it was summertime. I was kind of bored sitting around, so I went in charge of the second floor in the new building. I stayed there for a year, but in the meantime my engagement was broken off. It was crazy because we didn't even date or anything. I was upset so I left the General Hospital and decided to go to New York. I had a sister, Sheila, who was also a nurse, working at the General Hospital. She had graduated after I did. We both went off to New York in August of 1945.

"We went from St. John's to New York by boat. The day we arrived all you could see at the New York pier was ticker tape. It was absolutely wild! The war was over the day we arrived – the 15th of August. It was so exciting and everybody was going mad. It was great! I was delighted to be there. Fortunately, our cousin was there to meet us. I thought it was a gorgeous city. New York was a different place then. You could walk along the street by yourself. I never had any fear going into the city alone. It was a gorgeous place to go – go to the theater and do a lot of things.

"Our cousin lived on Long Island and my sister had stayed there when she went to university. My cousin had one child and her husband was dead, so it was a very good situation for us and for her. We knew it wouldn't be any problem to get a job because they were screaming for nurses. The papers were full of ads. We applied at several places, and everywhere we went, they asked if we brought our bags to stay. There was a hospital half a mile from my cousin's home. We started to work there as staff nurses fairly shortly after we arrived. We had no other special training or qualifications. I was on this huge floor, 45 patients. Sheila was put on a smaller floor. There was a terrible shortage of nurses and the nursing care really was appalling. I stayed there two weeks and thought, 'I can't work here under these circumstances.' There was no organization, no anything. This was a private teaching hospital and they were affiliated with a college. They had private, semi-private and four-bed rooms. Patient care was lacking; some got baths, some didn't; some beds were made, others weren't; some dressings were done and some weren't, and to me the whole thing was very unprofessional. So I went in to the Director of Nurses and said that I was sorry, I couldn't work under those circumstances. I didn't feel I could do a proper job in such a short time and everything was so sloppy. She begged me to stay, but I said, 'No, I'm sorry.' I went home and my sister Sheila said, 'Well, Mary, I have to work and I'm not going to stop. You have a few dollars but I don't have any.' The Director of Nurses called me at home and said she would have a Head Nurse's position open for me in two weeks if I would consider going back. She said, 'Please! You know, I was so impressed with what you told me, I figured you could run a very good floor. Give it another chance.' So I did.

"It was a small surgery floor but at least I was in control. I didn't have to listen to somebody else. When you were in control, you were able to make changes. There was a shortage of nurses but they had a lot of nursing assistants. You could show them how to do things and organize it so that the floor was run properly. I'd go around and see to the patients' needs. Shortly after I became Head Nurse another Head Nurse's position opened up and they gave it to my sister and we were fine. We worked on those floors for several years; I was there from '45 to '56.

"Then they asked me to take the position of Assistant Director of Nurses. I was in that role for two or three years when the Director of Nurses opened up and that's where I finished up. I really didn't want to take the position because I had no degree but there was such a shortage of nurses at the time that I had to. I even taught pediatrics at the college for a year. Even as Director of Nurses, I visited every patient in the hospital every day so that I knew what was going on. I had no trouble whatsoever. The staff was very cooperative. I was a stranger because they were all Americans and I was a Canadian, as they called me. I thought I'd have some reaction from some of the special nurses, Nassau Hospital graduates, but I didn't. Even when I became Director of Nurses, they were very supportive of me.

"I had to become an American citizen to write my State Boards examinations. You had to declare yourself willing to be a citizen before you could write those State Boards. *I was a Newfoundlander!* I was never a Canadian, but I did become an American citizen. I thought it only fair that I should. There were certain qualifications that I had to have. I got my marks from the General Hospital, but there were two subjects that weren't included in the curriculum so I had to be tutored for those and write the exams before I was allowed to write the State Boards. On top of that, they lost the exams I wrote so I had to write them over again, but I didn't mind.

"In 1956 I came home for a sister's wedding. I wasn't going to come home because I had a new apartment, had bought a lot of new furniture, and really couldn't afford the trip. But Sheila, who was married now, was coming and said, 'Come on.' So we came home and I met Doug. That was the 23rd of April. He had a car business. He came up the next month and asked me to marry him. I said, 'That's out of the question! I can't get married. I'm in a responsible position. I just can't go off and leave. At least I have to give them a couple of months' notice.' I resigned on the 15th of May and left the end of July, so it gave them a chance to get somebody else. We were married the 24th of August in New York.

"I still pay my fees in New York. I've always loved nursing and I still take an interest in it. I haven't nursed since I was married. I took care of my mother for seven years. Doug didn't want me to work after I was married and that's probably the reason why I didn't. But it was four years before I had a child so I did have lots of time to work. I still have a great love for it."

CHAPTER 14:

Marcella French

*"I always remember that was very important, the night
I got my cap… It was a big achievement. I felt more important
getting the cap than my pin and diploma."*

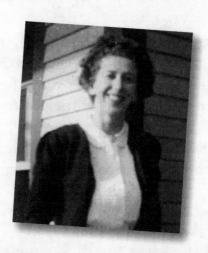

Marcella French was born in Bay Roberts in 1915 and graduated from the St. John's General Hospital in 1939. Shortly after graduation, she was admitted to the Sanatorium with tuberculosis of the lung. Upon discharge, she deferred her career to care for her mother who was disabled. She resumed nursing four years later when she took a position as staff nurse at the Sanatorium where she worked until her retirement.

Marcella grew up as an only child in French's Cove, a community of fourteen families. When she was 12, her family moved to Beachy Cove where she went to school until she was in grade 6. Then she moved to Bay Roberts. "It was great growing up in Bay Roberts. I don't ever remember being bored. We didn't have a load of toys, we just made our own. Being an only child was not good but I thought it was great up to about age nine or ten. The kids would say, 'You're lucky. You don't have to share,' and I thought, 'Maybe I am lucky.' But as I got a bit older, I realized I wasn't so fortunate. I realized as I grew up that other people's kids weren't always watched like I was. They had more freedom. I think my parents were overprotective.

"I had a job to get away when I decided to go into nursing. I just said, 'I'm going.' I don't know why I went into nursing. I wasn't very fond of kids for some reason so I figured I wasn't cut out to be a teacher. A couple of my friends went to a school on Springdale Street to do shorthand and typing but that didn't appeal to me. I could have stayed home until I was 95 before either one of my parents would have said, 'Are you ever going to do anything?' Finally I decided, 'This is it!' I was 21 and should have been finished with my training because they took them in at 18. I came into town one day and went down to the General and got an application form. I don't know why I chose the General, but actually I knew Pauline Sheppard and Kay Fraser, and they were in there. I don't know if that had any influence. When I went home and told my parents I was going into nursing, they just accepted it.

"I think we had to have two references. I got them from my teacher and the clergyman. We had to have ten uniforms, bibs and aprons. I had them made by a dressmaker in Bay Roberts. We wore pink uniforms at first and after our six-month probationary period, we wore pink stripes. They told you where to buy the material for the uniforms. We had to buy two pairs of special shoes from Parkers, but they were lovely shoes, very well made. We also had to have white stockings, a watch, and a pen. They even told us where to buy our scissors. It was all on the list they sent us.

"I loved the uniforms. As students, we wore a white bib and apron over the uniform. Then when we finished, we took off the bib and apron and got our black stripe. We wore a white uniform when we finished. The bibs and aprons were gorgeous, all starched and nice and clean. They weren't hard to wear except the collars and they weren't too bad. We had long sleeves and cuffs and when we went on duty, we'd take off the cuffs and roll up our sleeves. Our bibs and aprons went to the hospital laundry, but our collars, caps and cuffs had to go to the little Chinese laundry on Duckworth Street to get starched. We got them all done up for about fifteen cents and there was perhaps a half-dozen pairs of cuffs. The collars sometimes rubbed your neck, but you didn't go to the supervisor and say, 'I'm going to take this off. I'm not wearing it anymore.' You just wore it!

"They took a student into nursing training, as they needed a position filled. They called me and said, 'Report on a certain day.' Bessie Walsh and I happened to go in on the same day. Alice Bishop was a Nursing Sister and she was the one who took us in. She was great! She was my ideal of what a nurse should be. She was a typical nurse in my estimation – very professional, nice, kind and very helpful. I thought she was great!

"Bessie and I went in the last day of August. We had a strange class. We picked up three girls who came in the previous February. Then in September, we picked up three others for eight and then three more in November. I don't know how we managed with all the lectures we had. I don't know how the others caught up.

Miss Taylor, who was Director of Nurses, got sick about six months after we went in. Miss Mona Smith was the Associate Director of Nurses, and she did lectures, and Miss Mabel Smith was a staff grad on the ward. They took over and between the two of them, they took care of us. Just after we went in training, they had a graduation at Bishop Feild. Alma Mews was a music teacher and she had us singing and practicing for the graduation. It was a beautiful ceremony. But that was the last graduation until after we finished. I think there was a great upheaval when the director got sick.

"On our first day we were brought into the classroom and given a little talk. They used to post our names on the bulletin board, where we were to go to work. I was posted on Cowan Ward, which was very fortunate, because Miss Mabel Smith was one of the nicest supervisors and very understanding of your first day. She showed us around the ward. We were brought to the linen cupboard and told, 'Here's where we pack our linen.' I don't think we had much contact with the patients at this stage except to make the beds. But we were put on the wards right away that first day! We were scared stiff, afraid we were going to do something wrong. We were posted right away for classes. Miss Mabel Smith gave us General Nursing; Miss Leslie, the dietician, taught us at night after seven o'clock. We learned how to make little pats of butter to put on the private patients' trays. The private patients had menus to make out. We also had lectures from different doctors. We went to the university for chemistry and had our classes at night. We came off duty at seven o'clock in the evening, had to walk to the university on Parade Street, do our lectures, and be back by ten-thirty, no matter what. So we ran up to the university, did the lectures and ran home again to the General. There was no transportation but we didn't think that was terrible. I do now! But then we just accepted the rules. We had class after working nights. If you went to bed at nine in the morning and there was a class at 2 p.m., you were called at half-past one to go to class. It didn't matter that you just came off twelve-hour duty. When we had a class we wore our uniforms. I don't remember having time off except for one half-day a week.

"We didn't have any social life as a student. I used to go skating at the rink on Forest Road. We'd run to be home by ten o'clock when people made rounds. Some people would sneak out, but I didn't like to do that. I'd be scared to death.

"When I was in training I only got home on my vacation. We got one day once a month and a half-day each week. The only other time I went to Bay Roberts in my three years was when I worked in the OR and we got all day Sunday off. Marg King, one of the supervisors, said, 'I'm going to Brigus tomorrow on the bus. Why don't you come too?' I said, 'Okay,' and off we went in the morning. The taxi from Bay Roberts picked me up at the bus. That night when I went up to get the bus, it was gone and I was supposed to be to work Monday morning! This was tragic because then you didn't phone in and say, 'I've missed the bus and I can't get in.' I got a taxi back to St. John's so I'd be at work the next morning. Miss Mabel Smith called me to the office and said, 'My dear, don't you ever do that again. If you miss the bus, phone. Why didn't you call?' I said, 'But I was supposed to be to work Monday morning. I had to be to work!'

"As probies, we lived in Dr. Keegan's residence; his home had been turned into a nurses' residence. The third year we lived over in the new residence. There was a little room upstairs where the night nurses slept. We used to call it 'the dive.' If you were on night duty, you slept up there. There were two to four students in a room. The girls were nice; we were just like a family. You worked, studied, went to sleep, got up again and worked. The phone would ring at 6:00 a.m. and whoever answered it, called the others. We had breakfast at 6:30 and were on duty at seven o'clock. We had two hours off during the day but that was usually classroom time. The patients had already had their face and hands washed by the night nurses and had gone back to sleep for another couple of hours. We woke the patients up again to have their breakfast. There were twenty-three beds on a ward and two students made beds until they were finished.

"Complete bed-patients got their baths after their breakfast. Every bed-patient had a bath and clean linen every day. The up patients got their beds made as well but washed themselves in the bathroom. There were two supervisors on for the whole hospital. We got a report from whatever nurse was on each ward, which was usually a student. We got two or three patients each. There were usually two staff nurses on each ward, and they did medications. The senior students did dressings and compresses. It was the senior students' job every morning to prepare the dressing carriage that was on each ward, refill jars that needed to be refilled, and get the instruments sterilized. Sterilization was completely different because everything went to the OR to be sterilized.

"If you were on Sundays, there wasn't as much work with no doctors around, so we'd mend the rubber gloves with pieces from other gloves. Then they were packaged and sent to be sterilized. We'd cut gauze and make dressings that had to be folded properly. The grad on the ward showed us how to fold them. These were packaged and sent to be sterilized. We made up the dressing trays with the basins and bowls and then sent them to be sterilized. Then we would get a big bag of sterilized goods back from the OR. All solutions and the IV poles came from the OR. We'd have to stand up on a chair and pour it into the bottle.

"I enjoyed the probationary period even though it was difficult work. We really worked! We only did lectures in between times. You learned from experience then as much as you did from theory because we were put with the patients right away. In our first term, we did three months night-duty, seven to seven with no time off. When the six months was up, I was going on night duty one evening and Miss Mona Smith said, 'Come into the office for a minute, I want to give you your cap.' On my way on duty, I got my cap! That was my capping ceremony! I felt great! The cap meant a great deal because for six months during the probationary period you were always wondering, 'Am I going to make it?' I figured once I got my cap, that was it, I was accepted. That's how I felt about it. It was a big achievement. I felt more important getting the cap than my pin and diploma. My diploma was mailed to me in Bay Roberts and I don't know when I got my pin. I probably got it after I went back to work.

"I was a probie on Cowan Ward when a woman tried to commit suicide. She was a post-hysterectomy. She'd only been done a few days, and then patients were kept in bed for ten days post-op. I don't think they realized but it must have affected her psychologically. Isabel Kirby was the only nurse on the ward. She was behind the screen with the doctor looking after another patient. When she came out, she could hear screams. The doctor was gone. The patient across the way was awake and she said, 'Nurse, that lady just got out of bed and she's gone down that way.' Kirby went into the bathroom and looked all around but no sign of her. She called the supervisor and they searched around. The patient had climbed over the veranda off Cowan and jumped. That was a real tragedy! She survived but was an invalid because she did something with her back. She was moved to Alex and was still a patient when I graduated. Kirby was in a real state for a while but she got support from her superiors.

"We were going to go home the next day. I said, 'This is it! I'm not staying here any longer if this is what happens.' We weren't prepared for things like that and we had only been in a month.

Going to pack up and go! It was such a shock to us. You expect a patient to get better and go home. Oh, the innocence! In those days families accepted things. I never heard of any repercussions from the family. Luckily this other patient watched her go, realized she wasn't supposed to be out of bed and called the nurse. The patients were very good like that. They knew everybody's ailments: what was wrong and what wasn't wrong. On an open ward you had a better chance to see what's going on than in private rooms. It wasn't ideal because with twenty-three beds on a ward, there was no privacy, but they did have companionship. They looked out for the other patients because the nurse was alone and had responsibility for all the patients. If you needed help, whatever grad was on duty would usually come and give you a hand. When you had a big problem, I found they were always there and were willing to come.

"I remember my first encounter with death. I felt really sad about it because it was a girl about 18 or 19. She'd had an appendectomy with complications. We prepared patients for the morgue. If it was a male patient, the orderly prepared them. People went to their homes then rather than funeral parlours. We got them ready and if the patient was from any distance, we put them in the morgue until whoever came for them. We were always very careful to protect the other patients on the ward and put a screen around the bed. I don't think we told the patients about a death but I think they just knew. I think people accepted these things. Maybe it affected them to a certain extent, but not that it was detrimental to their getting better. I remember the horrible nitty gritty things about packing the patient. We packed the rectum but in the latter years that wasn't done by us; the undertaker did it. We closed the eyes and the jaw was bandaged and tied onto the end of the bed. We wrapped them in sheets but if they were going around the bay, we'd dress them in their clothing.

"We affiliated three months at the Grace, two months at the San, at the Mental, and two months at the Fever. We had a number of classes, but I always thought that when we affiliated at the Grace we should have gotten our obstetric lectures there and when we worked at the Mental, do our psychiatry lectures there. Instead we had to leave these places and walk back to the General for classes, and we also had to wear our street clothes for these outside classes. We had no taxis or anything so we used to thumb a ride. You didn't worry about people picking you up then, you just got aboard the first car that stopped. It could be rainy or snowy but you'd have to walk; it didn't matter. That was pretty rugged!

"I was on holidays when I was doing the obstetrics lectures. I had to come in from Bay Roberts three times in the three weeks of my vacation, because if you missed these lectures, you couldn't write your exam. I came in by taxi in the morning, did the lecture and went back by taxi in the evening for the three weeks. Those were the days! Class was on and you had to go! But all that changed when the director got sick and a new one came to the General to relieve; that was 1939 or '40. She was from somewhere on the mainland, but she changed things! She said it was absolutely ridiculous having girls out affiliating and not having a means of transportation back to class, so she employed one of the taxis in town. Maybe we didn't rebel against walking back to the General for class because we loved to go back there in the afternoon so we could stay for dinner. We thought the General had the best food. At the Grace, the VIPs had their own table and their own special food and the students didn't get that. The same way at the Mental. The grads had bacon and eggs but they fed us something different. But at the General, everybody got fed the same, from the VIPs down. Whatever one got, the other one got. So we were always delighted when we had classes in the afternoon! It was great! When we worked nights, we had to cook our own. The meals at the

General were quite good; they were nutritious.

"At the Fever there were about four or five grads. Patients in the Fever Hospital mostly had communicable diseases like diphtheria and typhoid. We had one patient in the iron lung; I think it was polio. We had to wear a gown, cap, and gloves when we went in to do the patients. We were given charge of two or three rooms over there; we didn't run from room to room. That was the only time we got two hours off during the night. We'd go out with the ambulance driver to pick up patients if they were suspected of having diphtheria or anything like that. Diphtheria was a big problem but we had our shots. I was never vaccinated for smallpox going in training, which amazes me. We were x-rayed on admission but then you didn't get x-rayed anymore unless you got sick, and there was a lot of TB around then. If someone came in with an appendix or any other illness and turned out to be positive for TB, it was called an open case. We also had patients on Victoria and Alexander Wards with draining sinuses, and a lot of these were positive for TB. I think this is why a lot of students caught it. I developed TB after I went to work as a grad, but there must have been four or five that got TB during training in the class behind me. It got so that it was frightening. Dr. Peters was furious! That's when they did something about it. After that, as soon as it was discovered there was an open case, everybody looking after the patient had to wear a gown and mask to protect themselves until the patient went to the San. But there was nothing like that when we were in training.

"During the probationary period, we were kind of on our own. We had great respect for all the people above us. It was a kind of a fear of the grads but with the directors, it was more respect. I never resented doing what I was told. If somebody told me to scrub the poles, I scrubbed the poles. That was part of the job. We didn't scrub floors; we had a few domestics on the ward who did that but we did the bathrooms. We had a few orderlies: Pat O'Reilly, Jim Gardiner and John Deere who were very good. They did catheterizations and things like that and were as good as half the grads.

"We had one emergency that I remember while I was in training. There was a mine explosion on Bell Island. I was in my third year. We had worked all day and we were asked to come back for a few hours to get the rooms set up for the patients because the few nurses on duty had their own work to do. There were seven or eight burn patients brought in. There weren't as many ORs as today and they could only do so much at a time. A couple of patients were put on Crowdy Ward, the surgical ward, and they worked on them there. That was really bad! Some were kept in the OR because there were no emergency rooms. There was a couple on Shea Ward, the medical floor, with severe burns. I remember one man whose fingers were just like bones, all scar tissue, and his face was all scar tissue. He was not nice to look at but you kind of got used to him. He had a lot of scar tissue because there was no plastic surgery then.

"I remember another burn case, an old lady with a big abdominal burn. They used a spray which caused a big black crusting and then it could heal from underneath. You had to watch that it didn't get septic underneath the big scab. One day I lifted it up and the veins and the arteries were exposed, but she survived. Then we used bakers' lamps. It was sort of like an igloo and you put it over the patient and turned on the lights for so many minutes. All the treatments were primitive compared to today.

"When we graduated, we didn't have a lot of expectations because there weren't a lot of opportunities. There were not a lot of positions for graduates. I had no idea where I was going to work so I went home after graduation. I thought, 'I need a rest. I need a month off at least.' I thought I'd write out a few applications but there wasn't much choice, only the few hospitals or health units outside. I thought, 'I'm just going to go to St. John's and live for a while.' When I went back to work, one of the girls and I talked about doing a PG [post graduate] at the Montreal General or the Royal Victoria. I think I would have done that if I hadn't gotten sick with TB. That changed my plans.

"I'd had an x-ray when I went to the San as a student because everybody was x-rayed when we went to affiliate and when we finished. Dr. Brown told me then my x-rays were perfect. But we had three years of hard work. One of the nurses from the General called me one day and said, 'Would you like to come back to the General? There's an opening if you want to come back.' I said, 'Yes,' and went back sometime in the spring. I had a cold, or so I thought, and got an x-ray. Dr. Brown said, 'I think you have some problems there.' I was devastated as I hadn't been back to work very long. I told Dr. Brown, 'I am not going to the San.' He said, 'Okay, child. Go home...then come back for another x-ray.' I'm not sure if he said six weeks or whatever. I was angry because I had just gotten back to work and now I was sick and all my plans were gone to pot. I didn't resent the system because I didn't have sense enough to know the system caused it. I didn't want to go to the San because you didn't know if you'd be there one year, five years or ten, but I was there from April until the following June. I had one tiny lesion, enough for me to have pneumothorax [collapsed lung]. I came out in June and Dr. Peters told me I could go back to work in October. Unfortunately my mother was ill with multiple sclerosis so I stayed home to care for her. I went back to work four years later. Dr. Peters used to visit and he'd say, 'Miss Wells wants you to come back to work.' And I'd say, 'I'm never going to work at the San!' Not that I disliked it; the people were great, but it wasn't what I wanted to do. I wanted to go to the Mental or the General Hospital. But Dr. Peters said, 'You can work with us at the Avalon Health Unit.' I said, 'No! I want to go work in St. John's.' Anyway I stayed home until my mother died and went back to work in May. I was really drained after my mother's death, so I thought, 'I'll go to work at the San,' never intending to stay. My father was on his own and the San was the nearest point where I could go back and forth by taxi (the story of my life!) until I bought a car and could drive home. It never bothered me about getting TB again; it's just that I didn't want to work there. I didn't have an application in, but Miss Wells called and told me they had vacancies and asked, 'Would you like to come back to work?' I said, 'Yes, I'd love to. Do you want me to make out an application?' She said, 'No, come on in.' I did the application after I went in. It was different then.

"We weren't allowed to accept monetary gifts but there wasn't much money floating around then. You didn't often get gifts but you didn't expect gifts either. Sometimes patients left bouquets or chocolates but usually they just said, 'Thank you.' Once in a while, you might get a pair of stockings. When I was in the San, there was a lady who'd bring something each time she came for a checkup. One morning she brought a bottle of smelts she had just done up that morning before she flew in. She said, 'Have them for your lunch now.' She was sweet!

"When I went in nursing my parents gave me to understand, 'If you go ahead with this, you do it right.' I don't ever remember feeling rebellious. We didn't ask, 'Why?' We just did it. But for all that I really enjoyed my training and I enjoyed nursing. I really did."

CHAPTER 15:

Gwen Thomas

"Nurse, you've got to come! You've got to come!"

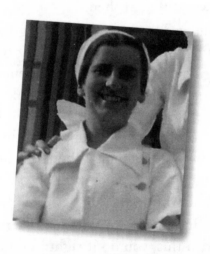

Gwen Thomas [Legrow] left South Wales and the V2 bomb in North London to accept the challenge of nursing in an outport in Newfoundland. She traveled to her patients by boat, plane, dog team, and komatik in all kinds of weather. The distances were often great, and she returned home only long enough to prepare for another call. The beauty of the country was her compensation.

When discussing her nursing school days Gwen Thomas recalled, "We went home when we had our time off, but we didn't have very much time off. We went on at seven o'clock in the morning and came off seven o'clock at night and then just didn't go anywhere. The Nurses' Home [residence] had very good facilities, I must say. We had a beautiful sitting room with a piano; we had records and we made our own fun and had lots of good times together. We all had our own room and they were well furnished. It was a new hospital and we were really well off.

"I always remember one particular night. I was a small person and they always took advantage of me. Everybody had a little clothes hamper in their rooms, and members of our class asked, 'Could you get in that clothes hamper? Are you small enough to get in that?' I said, 'I'll try.' So anyway they put me in the clothes hamper and dragged me out into the corridor. After a while the House Sister came along and said to them, 'What's that clothes hamper doing there in the corridor? You better take it back in the room straight away.' So the poor girls had to pick me up in the clothes hamper. They didn't say a word. There I was inside and heard this all going on! They took me right back to my room in the clothes hamper. And that was that. We had lots of fun!

"We had lovely Christmas concerts. We had all sorts of sketches and also a chorus line. I always used to kick up my legs in the chorus line. The seamstress at the hospital made all our costumes. We had a great time with lots of fun. I must say Christmas at the hospital was really something because about a month before Christmas, they'd have a fund for Christmas decorations. Each ward had a special theme for their decorations, especially the children's wards. A four-bed room on each ward was always kept vacant during Christmas and that was the social room. We had all kinds of goodies in this particular room and the doctors and nurses came to visit. We used to have really great Christmases!

We really did. I lived about five miles from home so I got home during Christmas. They used to get as many patients as possible discharged and we went all out for the patients who were left. And I must say the medical and the administrative staff went all out for the nurses too. The dinner was fabulous, there was nothing missing. The medical staff waited on us. They had everything so Christmas was really great.

"It was terribly hard work. You never stopped. Sometimes I'd go to bed at night so exhausted I could cry. The thing was, the Sisters wanted everything to be so perfect. For instance, the beds had to be just so. You had to have perfect corners, the sheets coming down nine inches over the mattress, and you had to have the pillows just so. When the matron came to do her rounds the patients were lying in bed like in a regiment, honestly. It wasn't the comfort of the patients, it was the perfection of the bed, and I'm not exaggerating. That's the absolute truth!

"One day another student and I had made all the beds on the older children's ward. The Sister came in and said, 'Humph! What's wrong with this bed?' She stripped them off and we had to make them all over again. When I think about it now, it seems unbelievable. The patients were well looked after but the regimentation was something else!

"As a probationer we gave the medications. We'd go around with the medications on the medicine trolley. The staff nurses checked every dosage and every medication before we gave it out.

"I worked with a patient with tuberculosis. In those days they had spooner mugs, little mugs that they used to spit into. We used to have to clean those out. The patients are sickest if they have hemoptysis [coughing blood]. And as they say, it was a poor town. A young boy died and that was the first time I had ever seen death. When I think about it, we were only 18 years of age and we were exposed to TB on that ward. They spit all over the place. I'm not exaggerating! Quite a few nurses contracted tuberculosis.

"I know the Sisters had a tough life too. I don't know what made the Matrons the way they were. The Sisters had to go to the Matron's office once a week for a meeting. I've seen them coming away from there completely devastated with tears in their eyes. It was the whole administration and it went down through the Sisters, the staff nurses, and the probationers, being the lowest of the low, had the brunt of it all. Seniority was very important. You'd have to experience it to understand. We'd go down to the dining room and as we went in through the door, if there was a probationer who started a month before you, she went in through that door first. If you were the last one accepted into that hospital you were the last one to go through that door and that's an absolute fact. If you just arrived at the school you just had to step aside while Sisters, staff nurses, third-year nurses, second-year nurses, all went in first. We didn't think about it really because our workday was so full. We accepted it all because it was part of becoming a nurse. You might think now and again, 'Well, gee whiz! Why should I put up with this?' but you had to accept things as they were. You couldn't think any less of yourself because of it. I was so naive in those days that honestly I didn't think we were being exploited. Now looking back on it, of course, we were. I often wondered about the Sisters because they became a Sister in the hospital and they were there for years and years and that was it. I don't remember very many of them having a life outside their profession. They were dedicated nurses and they might move to another hospital but most didn't.

"I was nursing at the beginning of the war. Even on our days off, if an air raid siren sounded, we would have to get up and go on duty to get the patients to the basement. Sometimes we were up half the night, as well as being on duty during the day. If I had some time off, I went home. Two of my brothers were home with my mother. Before we'd go to bed my mother said to me, 'If the siren goes tonight are you going to get up?' I said, 'No, indeed I'm not! I don't care if a bomb drops on me, I'm so tired.' So one of those times the siren went off, and we stayed in bed. All of a sudden we heard a loud ringing noise, like a bomb coming down. Well, it was a two-storey house, and we took shelter under the large dining room table. I don't remember how we all got downstairs, but the next thing I can remember was that EVERY one of us was under this table. It was just a small bomb that was dropped at the end of our road; you know it just made a hole.

"When I finished school, I went up to London and did the first six months of the midwifery courses at the London hospital. While I was there we had to go for lectures in public health as well as lectures in the hospital. When there was a delivery on our particular floor the bell would ring and the midwifery students and medical students would all rush to the caseroom to see the delivery. I will always remember one day, one of the patients was expecting twins so we were all very interested in the delivery and rushed to the caseroom. The medical students took turns with midwifery to do the deliveries. The medical student was ready to deliver the twins and we were all standing around the patient waiting. He was ready to catch the babies and the next thing we knew the first baby came out so fast it was as much as he could do to catch it before it fell in the pail! We were expecting a breach delivery but he didn't have to do a thing at all. He passed the baby to someone and there was the other baby. I'll never forget. I can still see him as a tall, dark thin fellow and the expression on his face when this baby arrived!

"For the second six months I went down to a maternity nursing home in Surrey. While there we did so much in the home itself and then so much out on the district. We used to go out on bikes with our little black bag. My first delivery by myself was in Surrey, because during our first six months we always had the teacher with us, but in the second part, they sent us out on our own. The baby was born. I just accepted it; it was just a normal thing. What amazed me was that the baby was 12 pounds! Most of the deliveries were in the home, rather than in the hospital. The family was there and we'd be with the mother for quite a while before the baby was born. We felt as if we belonged and they felt as if we belonged. Once the baby is born the first thing the mother would ask for was a cup of tea. We would make the mother and baby comfortable and do the baby up. The family would be so happy. It's a lovely feeling! If a patient has good antenatal care I think a home delivery is an excellent thing. The babies were delivered when the babies were ready. We weren't allowed to use forceps to force the baby out. Sometimes we were allowed to do episiotomies. I have done that but I never did it very often. I guess because we waited and allowed them time to deliver.

"The doctor who was there at that particular time was one of the pioneers of painless childbirth. He'd give the patients breathing exercises and educate them about what to expect next. He'd calm them down and it was amazing. I must say in this nursing home in Surrey the care was the epitome of childbirth. I think that this second six months of my midwifery training taught me how important it is to look after the mother beforehand.

"I was in London for the last year of the war when they sent over the V1 and V2. That was frightening because you never knew whether they were going to drop. It's amazing how everyone just went on living, went and did their daily job. The fact is that it brought people closer together. The V2 bombs were the bombs that you couldn't hear. There would be terrible explosions and devastation. This particular morning I went on duty in the nursery. Well when I went in, there were pieces of the wall gone, pieces of the ceiling down. One of these bombs had fallen in a factory across the road, and it had done some damage to the hospital itself.

We always kept mesh over the babies' cots for protection. The pieces of plaster came down on the mesh but none of the babies were hurt. The morning after the V2 fell I was called to do a cauterization on a wound. I put the screen around the patient and put on my gown and gloves. After I finished I came out and the ward was in a mess with plaster everywhere. More plaster had fallen from the ceiling.

"I can't remember exactly how many babies I delivered but from 1945 to 1949 that's all I did. It was quite a few hundred. Prenatal care was the important thing and if we expected a problem the obstetricians and gynecologists were the right people to look after these particular patients. If there were no complications we looked after them. They had confidence in us and we stayed there with them. I think anyone in childbirth needs somebody with her, as a comforting presence.

"When I worked at the L. B. Hospital we had a patient who must have been in her early 40s because she had two children, one was 18 and the other was 20. She was in the caseroom and we were expecting twins. It was a routine delivery. We delivered the first baby, a fine little boy, and the second baby, another little boy; he was fine. I was looking after the two babies and the assistant nurse was with the mother waiting for the afterbirth. She said, 'Sister, Sister, there's another baby.' I said, 'Go on!' So I went up, and true enough, there was another baby boy. She had triplets. They were about five pounds. What a shock it was for the mother!

"I enjoyed midwifery the most, especially the home deliveries. If I hadn't come to Newfoundland, that's where I would have stayed! After the war the Overseas Nurses had this ad and it said that nurses were wanted in Bermuda and Newfoundland. I didn't know anything about Newfoundland so I sent in an application for there. I thought it would be a challenge. I had to go to a Harley Street doctor for a medical examination and the doctor said, 'Yes, nurse, you're A-One. You're really healthy. You're okay to go to Newfoundland.' I came and enjoyed it.

"When I went to La Scie, it was 1949, and there was a lot of tuberculosis in Newfoundland. In quite a few families, one person or another was in bed with TB and eventually died. At that time they used to have special relief for the TB patients. I used to have to go Shoe Cove quite a lot, and to Brads Cove. In the winter we would go by dog team and in the summer we'd go by boat. My district was Round Harbour and as far as Pacquet. Mostly I used to go to those places by boat; one time I did walk to Round Harbour but never to Brads Cove. The only way to get into La Scie was either by plane or in the winter by dog team, in the spring and summer by boat, or else across the woods roads.

"I remember one time going to Shoe Cove, which was about four and a half miles, and we had to walk because there were no roads. When I arrived, the patient was in labour. She had twins, which I delivered. Later that evening I began walking back to La Scie. I got back about a mile, I guess, and they came running after me. She was bleeding and was a pretty sick women. I could see her getting paler and paler. I thought there was no good trying to get any help; I mean, where was I going to get help? So I raised the foot of the bed and I put in packing and I gave her procaine. I did all I possibly could, and I said to her husband, 'I can't do anymore. I'm sorry!' Then all of a sudden it stopped and she didn't bleed anymore. I don't know why. I thought I was going to lose her. She really gave me quite a scare.

"I always remember the dental experience I had at La Scie. We used to pull teeth in those days and I came to St. John's for three weeks of orientation. We went to Dr. Hogan's clinic to learn how to pull teeth. He had forceps and a kidney dish and he was so fast pulling teeth that I was afraid. I went out to La Scie with only an upper jaw and a lower jaw forceps. That was it! Of course there was no dentist at that time. The dental experience I had was practically nothing and I'm telling you Newfoundlanders' teeth are hard! My sister was a public health nurse in London and she did dental clinics. One day, she told the dentist that her sister was out in Newfoundland and extracted teeth. And he said, 'What? Extracts teeth? Heavens, I was in the navy during the war and those Newfoundlanders had the hardest teeth. Their teeth are just like rocks! They're the hardest teeth to pull!' I had an ordinary kitchen chair, and the jaw forceps, and Novocain. Anyway, there was one family in La Scie and there were quite a few boys in the family. The boys would go out in the woods, and they were really tough, hard workers. One day one of them came and wanted his tooth pulled, so I gave him the injection and waited. Then I put the forceps on and tried to pull it and he passed right out. He was really one of the tough ones, but he passed out!

"The funniest thing of all happened the first year I was in La Scie. The mail came by dog team from Nippers Harbour. The mail carriers were brothers, and they were both six-foot tall, both fine men. One of them came to the clinic and said, 'Nurse, I have a terrible tooth. You have to get the tooth out,' It was one of his back teeth so I sat him in the chair and gave him the injection and I waited. When I started to pull, well, it was like trying to pull out a rock! I could not move it. 'I can't get that out,' I said. But he said, 'Yes, you have to get it out. I've been tormented for too long.' I said, 'Look, you have to go over to Twillingate.' 'No,' he said, 'you've got to have that tooth out this afternoon! You and I are going to get this tooth out!' So I hauled and hauled; the more I pulled, the more he moved down in the chair, and the next thing I knew he was lying on the floor. Then I straddled him and put my hand over the forceps and he put his hand over mine and eventually, between the both of us, we got it out. He was so desperate!

"I'd go to Brads Cove by dog team. The hill going through the community was so icy that they would always tie me onto the collar tip, in case I'd fall off. I was like a lamb led to slaughter! Once I was on the collar tip, I could not get off unless they took me off. We got to the brow of the hill and the dogs had so much momentum we went right down though the community, right out onto the frozen harbour. We could not stop! There I was on the komatik and the poor old dogs dragging behind me. The driver had jumped off. Usually he just stood on the back of the sled but he couldn't hold the force.

"I treated a lot of pneumonia, a lot of bowel trouble, pains in the stomach, and so forth, coughs, flus, and quite a few accidents. There was one particular accident in La Scie involving a fisherman. Fishermen used to boil bark for dipping their nets and they would have the pot covered. One of this man's legs went right into the boiling bark and the other one partly in. All the skin was scalded, and his legs were in pretty bad state. He was a lovely person, in his 50s. I told him the best thing to do is to go to Twillingate. 'No, Nurse,' he said, 'you look after me. I don't want to go over there.' He would have to wait for the coastal boat to come or go over on a fishing boat. He said, 'I don't want to leave home, you can look after me.' I treated him with sulpha ointment and eventually it healed after about three months. I guess he must have been a pretty healthy type. I'd go in about twice a week to see how he was getting on. I guess it was painful, but he didn't complain.

"I was the first nurse in La Scie to use penicillin. It was a godsend for pneumonia! We had patients terribly sick with pneumonia. First when I went there, all we had were the sulfa drugs. If there were anything that I felt was beyond my capacity, I'd get a plane or boat and send them to Twillingate or St. Anthony. I did a lot of simple surgery, but when it came to surgery for broken bones, or something that I'd never done before, I'd send them off.

"What used to tickle me was that they would come to the door and say, 'Nurse, you've GOT to come!' Not 'Will you?' 'You've GOT to come!' regardless of the time of the day. I remember one winter night about twelve o'clock, there was a heavy snowstorm. A man came over from Pacquet and said, 'We've got a young man that is very sick. Will you come?' So I went on this little boat; it had a little house on it. We were about four hours on the water, and there was a priest aboard. He was a very nice person, but all the way across he kept telling me how good I was to get out at night and how the good Lord would look after me and that sort of thing. I thought, 'Gee whiz! I wish I wasn't here.' We got across and it was snowing, so we could hardly see where to get into Pacquet. We saw the light and went up to the house. There was a young man about 30 dying with TB. All I could do for him was make his end a little bit easier. He was really frightened. It was a terrible experience, facing that young man.

"One time I had a call from Brads Cove. I was due to leave on a holiday that evening. The boat was coming in so I went and there was a little boy that had a prong from a fishhook through the middle of his hand. There were all of these people in Brads Cove and they couldn't do anything! Well at least they thought they couldn't. They had to get the nurse. The little boy was around nine years of age and he had a small thin hand. The only thing to do was to file through the jigger. So I filed it. I gave him something to apply to the wound and I left some dressings. I was away for about two weeks and when I went over to see the little boy it had healed over. What amazed me was how the people didn't have the presence of mind to file it off. For a while in La Scie, they were without a nurse, but once one came, the nurse had to cure them. In some cases it was psychological. You'd give them something and they'd think they were better. Of course, it wasn't all like that. There were genuine cases that had to be looked after and sent to hospital, but sometimes people need somebody to give them a little confidence.

"I got married in La Scie around eight o'clock in the evening. The people in the community came to the wedding and reception. My vacation had started but we had to wait a couple of days for the coastal boat to come before we could leave. When you're in an outport your vacation doesn't start until you've left the community. We stayed at the boarding house and around about five in the morning there was this bang on the door. I always knew, when there was a bang on the door in the night, that I was the one that was wanted, so I went down. It was a girl having her first baby and she was in labour. My husband didn't say a word. Off I went and I was there from five until eight o'clock in the morning. I delivered the baby boy and the mother was okay. After that, I walked back to where we were staying and got back into bed with my husband. That was our wedding night! Not very many people would go to a maternity case on their wedding night.

"We had no family in La Scie and there were only a few friends where we dined and played cards. There was a teacher who was in the Royal Air Force before he was a teacher. We got to know them very well. There were quite a few other families that we mixed with socially. They were really intelligent. I think they knew more about things than I did. There were quite a few families there that I respected.

"I was too busy to go to the 'Times' [community parties] because I was away a lot to the other communities. When I was back I wasn't too interested in going out to functions. All I wanted to do was relax. I read a lot. I had books sent to me from the Newfoundland Library. I had the radio and I did a lot of embroidery work. We also went into the country a lot, especially with one family we were very friendly with. We'd go fishing with them and have lots of picnics. We enjoyed outdoors a great deal.

"I was brought up Methodist and there was a United Church

in La Scie. I used to go to church every now and then, but sometimes I'd go fishing on Sunday. Some thought my friends were leading me astray. They didn't realize that I loved being out in the country where there were beautiful ponds. We'd go out codjigging, boil up fish and brewis on the beach and that sort of thing. I always liked berry picking. Those are the nice things I remember about the country.

"After La Scie we moved outside St. John's and I went to work at the Janeway. I was a staff health nurse. I got to know all the staff, from the kitchen staff to the administration. That's what I liked about the Janeway. I worked as the staff nurse and was involved with the whole of the hospital. I meet some of them every now and then, and I'm really happy to see them because I feel as if I know them. Staff would all come to me for their immunizations and of course, their chest x-rays and that sort of thing. I used to look after the different lab tests that they used to undergo. It was a job in general health care. I really enjoyed my days down at the Janeway.

"I also worked a little while in Emergency and Outpatients in the Janeway. In Outpatients, all you did was take the chart to the doctors, who would examine the patients, and then you'd have to see that whatever the doctor ordered would be carried out. It wasn't bedside nursing care. It was completely different. Of course La Scie wasn't bedside nursing care either. The only bedside nursing care that I did was in my early days during training. I think that I'd rather be out in public health rather than on the ward with bedside nursing. That's more my way."

Helen D. Penny

"I always thought team nursing was practiced long before the team nursing we later came to know. There was a bonding between nurses; one helped the other. We'd go on those big wards in the morning and…each would take one row of patients. The nurse finishing first automatically helped the others. That's how we got through."

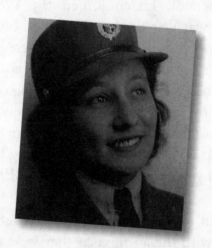

Helen D. Penny was born in English Harbour in 1920. She did aerial photography during World War II before going to nursing school. She graduated from the General Hospital School of

Nursing in 1949 and completed a post-graduate course in public health at the University of Toronto. She returned to the General Hospital, assuming the positions of teacher to Associate Director. In 1961, Miss Penny accepted the challenge of Director of Nursing at the new hospital in Grand Falls, and under her leadership, the hospital received full accreditation within one year of opening.

Helen Penny spent her early childhood in New York where her father had gone to work. When she was 12 her family returned to Newfoundland, as her father's health deteriorated and he wanted to come back to Newfoundland to have surgery. The family lived in English Harbour for a year or two following their return, but as it was remote from St. John's and a lot different from New York, they moved to Hants Harbour, which was the home of Miss Penny's mother. She remained there until she completed school.

After high school, Helen joined the Women's Division of the RCAF. "It was war time and I joined before I went into nursing. Newfoundland was a country then so I went with '*Newfoundland*' on my shoulder badge. Half a dozen of us went from Newfoundland. We did our basic training outside Ottawa. I did my photography training in Moncton, New Brunswick, and did aerial photography in the air force. We were the only air force girls who flew, so it was interesting and exciting times. I stayed in over two and a half years and was discharged in 1945 when the war was over.

"I had decided to go in nursing before I left the air force. I was asked to stay with the air force as they were starting an aerial survey of the north and wanted some of the photographers to stay on a permanent basis. I had applied for nursing in Toronto and in St. John's. The new General Hospital on Forest Road was just opened and my mother sent me the newspaper clippings. I weighed the pros and cons and thought, 'I'll go back home.' My mother was very happy! I entered nursing in February 1946 and graduated in 1949. It was easier for me to adjust to nursing because of my military background, but even if I had gone in cold, I think I had the advantage of being a little more mature. It was easier to meet and relate to people having worked with people from many places inside and outside of Canada.

"As a student I lived in the residence attached to the old wing of the hospital. You came through the tunnel and the school was in the basement. We had twelve-hour days as a student, six days a week, with Sundays off, but it wasn't very long before your Sunday off disappeared. You were lucky if you got a half day once every few weeks.

"After six months we received our caps and started clinical practice in the hospital, although we did quite a bit of clinical practice during our first six months. It was so different in so many ways, the types of care required on a large ward like Carson. We had all types of cases in the one area. I remember we had a 16-year-old girl on Victoria ward dying of tuberculosis and then we had a man admitted with syphilis. If you had TB patients you did everything: sterilized their dishes, bedpans, and the utensils they used, and disposed the remnants of their food in the utility room. Tuberculosis was prevalent in our day. A couple of girls in my class contracted it and didn't finish nursing. Several others were treated at home after a short period in the Sanatorium. They came back after two years or so and completed their nursing. We did a lot to avoid contracting TB; we gowned, masked, and scrubbed and used a lot of alcohol on our hands and arms.

"I was a patient in hospital for three weeks with rheumatic fever. There was one night-nurse on the second floor who would rush up and down the corridor all night. You could hear the rustle of her starched uniform. She never stopped. It was a rush against time! There was only 12 hours and you were responsible for 20 to 30 patients and everything went through your hands. When this nurse came in to me, I said, 'That's an awful colour you have,' and she'd say, 'Penny, I've had it for ages.' On the morning I was discharged from hospital I went back to the residence. I wasn't over there very long when the Director of Nursing phoned and told me to report for duty on that floor. No such thing as time to recuperate! I was informed that the nurse who had been on duty that night was transferred to the Sanatorium that morning. She was not in very good condition. I went to the second floor that evening and took her place. You didn't question or say, 'Why can't we have more people?' The people weren't available. That's why you didn't go off ill because if you did you were going to be missed and someone was going to have to work twice as hard.

"Nursing was hard work and we didn't have the auxiliary help that is available today. Different kinds of work went through the one pair of hands. You cleaned medicine cupboards every day and removed everything to clean. You cleaned your patient's locker and drawers. There were so many things that had to be done. The nursing assistants had a handful of patients and there were a couple of senior orderlies, but the nursing staff carried out all the responsibilities. Hard work and long hours may have contributed to some nurses' illness but surprisingly it was all right: the work, the long hours and the demands. There was always the constant stress you could be exposed to TB or something, but there wasn't much grumbling or complaining. I always thought team nursing was being practiced long before the team nursing we later came to know. There was a bonding between nurses; one helped the other. We'd go on those big wards in the morning and each of us would take one row of patients. The nurse finishing first automatically helped the others. That's how we got through.

"Occasionally, we would get male patients from the penitentiary. A police car would come screaming up to the admitting entrance with the inebriated from downtown. If the guards didn't come we were responsible for them. You'd put them on a stretcher between other patients because there were no empty beds. If they were drunk and noisy it was distressing for other patients who should be getting their sleep. Some weren't noisy; they would just sleep it off. In the mornings we'd get them on their way again. We had the task of trying to clean them up and many of them needed to be cleaned. I remember using chloroform on a patient because soap and water just wouldn't do it.

"One female patient came in on a regular basis and one morning I said to her, 'If you come in like this again I don't know what I'm going to do with you.' She talked loudly and could be a bit boisterous. I remember her because she was murdered later on. She had two children, a boy and a girl. As far as I was concerned, she was more sinned against than sinner. She was never married and an avid smoker. Alcohol brought so much unpleasantness to her life. She didn't know how to cope. She came in one time when I was on Carson and had her leg amputated. She was a difficult patient but if you ignored it you could handle her without any problem. I always did her dressings and afterwards I'd stay with her so she could have a cigarette. She spent her life fighting everybody when what she needed was someone to care.

"We had a few patients with typhoid fever in those days. Pneumonia was also a major problem but cancer was just not as prevalent then. We'd see a few old gentlemen with cancer of the lip from smoking a pipe. Mastectomies and other types of cancer surgery were few and far between. There was a lot of corrective surgery for women, which I thought was due to the lack of good prenatal care. There was no pill in those days and birth control was not practiced like it is today. Women had large families and were sadly neglected.

"I was on night duty as a float nurse and went to Victoria ward to relieve the nurse for an hour. She was a classmate of mine. When I arrived, she said, 'You've come to a poor place tonight. There are three patients dying and they could die while you're here.' I had never seen a dead person until then. She briefed me and I took over the ward. A young woman in her late twenties was dying from TB. I phoned Miss Feehan, the night supervisor, and told her time was running out fast. She came right away and the patient died while we were both there. We laid her out, dressed her in her wedding gown and veil, which her husband had brought in that night. He knew she was dying and left them for us. She was so emaciated. It was the saddest thing. I thought it was inappropriate to lay her out in her bridal attire because as a bride she must have looked a lot different than she did that night. That was the first patient I ever helped to prepare after death. That was a traumatic experience!

"I had a lot of memorable experiences on Victoria ward. We got a lot of patients with lice. I remember one woman came in midmorning. She had a lump on her forehead and was running an elevated temperature of 106! I told the nurse in charge and she called the doctor. When the doctor came, he asked for a tray, which I prepared and then assisted him. He incised the lump and it was a lice bag. It just came pouring out! I had never seen anything like it before. She recovered but was a very sick girl for a while.

"When on night duty, nurses slept in the night nurses' residence, which at the General Hospital was located in the old orthopedic residence. A classmate and I were on night duty and sharing a room. In those days we were on night duty three months at a time. On one of our nights off, we went to see a movie, which was a treat because we so seldom got the opportunity. When we came back and went to bed, Ruth was tossing and turning in her bed. I said, 'What's the matter? You are restless tonight.' She said, 'Aren't the mosquitoes bothering you? They're playing havoc with me.' I said, 'No, I don't feel any mosquitoes.' I heard her slapping herself and could see her white arms going. She said, 'It's getting worse. I'm being devoured by mosquitoes.' I said, 'Turn on the light and let me see. I'm not bothered at all. Your blood must be sweeter than mine.' I turned on the light and went to look. I pulled back the bedclothes; she was bitten and blood everywhere. I had never seen any before but it came to me in a flash. I said, 'Ruth, you're not being bitten by mosquitoes. It's bedbugs.' I called the residence director, who came, took one look, and called the night supervisor at the General, who brought the doctor. Ruth was whisked away to the General and I was whisked out of the room. They fumigated everything. I was working at the Fever Hospital and felt really depressed having to go back to that room. It wasn't funny but memorable!

"We had all kinds of patients at the Fever Hospital, from babies to adults. That was the only time I was ever hit by a patient. He was a young man diagnosed with meningitis. The doctor came to do a spinal tap and I had set up the tray for him. We turned the patient on his side in the proper position. Just as the doctor was going to insert the needle, without any warning, the patient came out of bed with his arm up and took one swipe. He sent the doctor and me flying. He hit me in the side of head and I literally saw stars! The tray, everything, went flying but he was not really responsible.

"When I was a young nurse on Alexander ward, we had small children, infants to maybe 18 months old. There were a couple of rooms at the back of the ward, one for post-op tonsillectomy and another room. I was on nights and we had a young woman, from the penitentiary, who was covered from head to toe in a syphilitic rash. It was the first and only syphilitic rash I ever saw. I've never forgotten it! My first thought was 'My technique has to be focused tonight with the babies and a post-tonsillectomy patient to care for along with a patient with a syphilitic rash.' Penicillin was just coming into its own and when I gave that patient her 6 a.m. penicillin, there wasn't one bit of rash on her. It was so strange! Penicillin was called the wonder drug, and for staff and patients it was. It made such a difference.

"We affiliated at the Waterford Hospital, and the General students stayed on the top floor in a three-storey house. There were five of us sharing one big room. This Saturday night it was blowing a gale like St. John's gets sometimes. We were in bed but one of the nurses was coming back from the bathroom. She turned to go to her cubicle when the big plate glass window blew in. If it had hit her, it would have cut her horribly! The glass went all over the room but none of us were injured, we just ducked under the bedclothes. If home had been nearer I guess that's one time we might have gone home.

"In one hospital where we affiliated, I saw a tremendous difference between the kind of care given to the rich as opposed to that given to the poor. It was noticeable to me from the beginning. The patients of means received more care and attention than those on the ward. I enjoyed my time there but I couldn't accept that. There was such a distinction between private and ward patients; the food, the presentation of it, the tray, even the china was different. From my observation, the nurses in that hospital seemed to do quite a bit of catering. I believe that a patient is a patient and all patients should receive the maximum care they require. You should give as much of your time, care, and sensitivity to a patient who is not as well endowed with worldly goods as some others. At the General Hospital we did not have many private rooms until we got the new wing. I always thought that patients on the ward received as good care as patients on the third floor in a private room.

"An uncle of mine was rushed to hospital by ambulance

from Hants Harbour while he was on holiday from New York. The doctor came by ambulance with him and he was in very poor condition. They called me to say they were bringing him in and I alerted Admitting. Mrs. T. said, 'Do you want to put him up on the third floor in a private room?' I said, 'No, I want him on Shea ward.' That's where they put him with special nurses. I knew he would receive the best of care there. The patients were under observation all the time. You couldn't walk down the corridor without observing twenty-one patients. The only thing missing on the wards was privacy.

"It was an exciting era with the introduction of penicillin and drugs for tuberculosis. When I worked at the Sanatorium, it was amazing to see all the young men and women and very young children there. On my ward there were two brothers in the same room; one in his twenties and the other only nine years of age. We also had a lot of men from the mines in St. Lawrence. I went to work at the Sanatorium in 1950 and left late in 1951 or '52. I thought if I stayed there any longer, I wouldn't want to leave because you get very attached to patients you care for over a long period of time. The administrator, Dr. Bennett, wanted me to do post-graduate work and come back to the Sanatorium. I wanted to do post-graduate work but the Sanatorium was not where I wanted to spend my time in nursing. I knew I had to uproot myself and leave.

"When I was at the Sanatorium we did a lot of things because there was no housekeeping staff and we did what had to be done. It was when team nursing came into play. The nursing assistants and orderlies were marvelous and very committed to patient care. We would talk about how we could improve the environment where the patients lived. The floors were wood, and though they were cleaned and scrubbed, they always looked dingy. We ordered the first wax ever used on the floor in the Sanatorium. It made them look bright and better and gave the patients a lift. We had a housecleaning routine; we did the rooms, the walls, the fixtures, everything. When I went there, I looked at the light fixtures and they were full of flies! The windows were wide open, summer or winter. Dr. Miller came in one afternoon to make rounds after the staff had done the fixtures. After he left, Dr. Bennett came back and said to me, 'Dr. Miller was very impressed with the ward. The things he noticed, you wouldn't believe! He wanted to know how come the fixtures on your ward were so clean and the others full of flies. He noticed your floors and the surroundings and I wanted you to know.' I thanked him.

"You really didn't expect pats on the back as a nurse but sometimes you did get them from unexpected sources, a patient or an understanding Head Nurse or supervisor. You were evaluated and the evaluations I saw were fair. If there was criticism, it was usually constructive. There are individuals in nursing who should never have been in nursing, but you get them in every walk of life. Some nurses you liked and greatly respected but I remember a couple that I found very difficult to respect. There was one nurse ahead of me who I thought was excellent. If I had a role model it was her. There were other good nurses but there was something special about her.

"Sometimes I felt I had power as a nurse, but I think I had the greatest control during my years at Grand Falls. There I was in the position to really exert influence on the ward. The board that directed the hospital was marvelous. They were all men but they listened to my point of view as the Director of Nursing as much as they did to the administrator. I had a great deal of respect. I was able to do things that I was never been able to do before and had a freer hand. It was satisfying to go to a new hospital, helping to formulate policies and select staff. They were very challenging years. I went with some reluctance because I felt the winds of change were coming in nursing. I do not have a degree in nursing, something I have always regretted. I thought a new hospital should have a director more academically qualified than I was. I never applied. I was approached. I declined at first but was invited to come out and look at the hospital with no strings attached. I couldn't. The Chairman of the Board reassured me they had a number of applicants with degrees apply for the job, both from outside Newfoundland and a couple from within. He said I had something they wanted at that particular time. I didn't make up my mind then and came back to St. John's. If I had not accepted the job I would always think that maybe I was afraid to take the challenge. I accepted the appointment. I've never had any regrets! It was a big challenge, opening a new hospital. I was there six months before it opened, ordering equipment and planning stage by stage. After the opening, we decided to go for accreditation in the first year of operation. We thought we had to be accredited as quickly as possible in order to get the kind of staff to give the quality of care we wanted. We got the staff together, told them what we wanted to do and what would be involved for them and for us because they were going to have to do a lot of hard work. Everyone was for it, and again it was a team effort. When we achieved accreditation, it was one of the greatest feelings of satisfaction I've ever had in my nursing career. It was tremendous! The surveyor was from Quebec. He said when he heard he was going to a hospital in Newfoundland that was opened only one year, he thought we must have bats in our heads. He came to my office that evening before he left and said, 'Miss Penny, people have achieved an awful lot here in a short time, such as policies and procedures in the nursing department. I'm the administrator of a hospital that has been opened eight years. We still do not have some of the things you have here.' I felt that was quite an accolade. We opened June of '62 and got accredited in 1963. It wasn't me but a marvelous staff working together. I was very fortunate to have the people I had working with me. It wasn't easy to uproot myself from the

General but it was good preparation. Without it I couldn't have taken on that job.

"I'm definitely glad I was a nurse. I think unless a young woman really wants to be a nurse, really has a feel for it, she should stay out of it. When I went into nursing there weren't as many avenues open to young women as there are today. Photography was fine for wartime. I was always interested in political science and law, but I am not sure if these were available at the time, whether my life would have gone in another direction."

Conclusion

At the time of these interviews nurses functioned more like physicians or the nurse practitioners of today, often because of their isolation. In fact, when the physician entered the nurse's territory there were frequently conflicts over ownership of the practice. Today the opposite can be seen as nurses learn advanced skills that allow them to cross over into traditional doctors' practice territory, and again conflicts arise.

Out-migration from Newfoundland and Labrador is a worrying trend now, as it was when these women were interviewed, even though many see it as a new movement in today's world. A nursing career still offers the option of travel and adventure to young people. Nursing skills vary little worldwide, although the geography, culture, and politics change. Young people will always seek new adventures, and nursing is a career that allows for travels and new experiences.

A welcome change has been the introduction of men into nursing. Men have brought their own perspectives to the practice of nursing, and nursing is the better for including them. However, looking back over the stories of the early nurses gives us a glimpse at what the lives of women were like back then and adds the female perspective to history in Newfoundand that most often recorded only the achievements of men.

These women lived at a time when they were not expected to go outside their own community and class. Ambition and curiosity about the world were seen as male traits, yet these women had both, and using nursing as the vehicle, they made their mark in history. They probably thought their stories held nothing unusual. Many unrecorded nurses could tell stories such as those included here. It is important that we ensure that their narratives are collected as well to preserve the history of nursing.

Nursing interviews today would relate stories showing a completely different set of nursing skills involving more technology and a greater ease with communication. There is far less isolation. The science and art of nursing has changed over the years, but the nurse's dedication to the patient remains the same.

Acknowledgements

We would like to acknowledge the Smallwood Foundation Research Grant, awarded in 2005, and the Association of Registered Nurses of Newfoundland and Labrador Violet Ruelokke Research Grant, awarded in 2003. These grants made it possible to have the nurses' interviews transcribed.

We also thank Joanne Smith-Young at the Memorial University School of Nursing Research Unit for her expertise and care in transcribing the interviews used in this book.

Jeanette Walsh 🙰 Marilyn Marsh 🙰 Marilyn Beaton

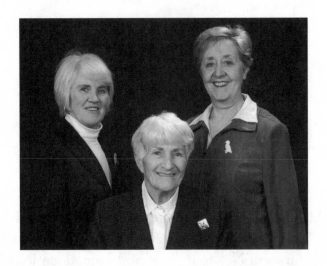

Marilyn Marsh RN, BN, MEd

Marilyn Marsh is retired from nursing after a 35-year career in the profession. She worked as the Nurse-in-Charge at the Sunshine Camp, Children Rehabilitation Centre, as well as taught at Memorial University School of Nursing for 28 years. During this time Marilyn was also involved in professional activities at both the provincial and national level. Because of her keen interest in preserving the history of nursing, Marilyn collected these stories. She is a volunteer at the Lillian Stevenson Archives/Museum preserving nursing history.

Jeanette Walsh RN, BN, MScN

Jeanette Walsh is retired from nursing after a 35-year career in the profession. She worked in a variety of nursing positions but spent the majority of her career in nursing education, primarily at the General Hospital School of Nursing. During this time Jeanette was also involved in professional activities at both the provincial and national level. She comes from a family tradition of nursing, with her sister, aunt and several cousins in nursing. Jeanette volunteers at the Lillian Stevenson Archives/Museum preserving nursing history.

Marilyn Beaton RN, MScN, MBA
Professor, School of Nursing
Memorial University of Newfoundland

Marilyn Beaton has been a nurse for 38 years. For 35 of those years she has taught at the Memorial University School of Nursing. Throughout her career she has been active in nursing, serving on various provincial and national committees. Marilyn comes from a family tradition of nursing, with her mother, aunt and sister all nurses. Because of them and all the nurses she has met, she wanted to preserve the stories of the nursing profession. She is presently working with Jeanette Walsh on a third project on the history of nursing.

From the Voices of Nurses

MARILYN BEATON & JEANETTE WALSH

"...a confirmation and celebration of the service and duty chosen by so many women... It gives us the flesh and blood realities of a demanding profession..."

– Jocelyne Thomas, *The Current*, September 2004

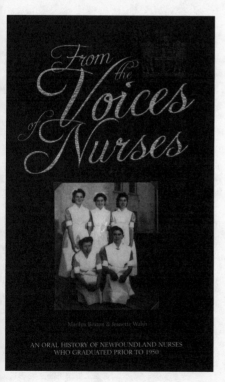

Thirty-three nurses who graduated before 1950 were interviewed about nursing in communities throughout Newfoundland and Labrador. Their experiences and stories reflect the nurses' perceptions and feelings about the nursing school experience, practicing nursing in various settings and communities, and the changes in the nursing profession throughout their careers. The stories also give insight into the commitment and strength of a generation of nurses.

ISBN 978-1894377-10-2 $14.95 PB

Available through the publisher and at fine book stores.